Becoming Certified in Neurofeedback:

A Guide to the Neurofeedback Mentoring Process for Mentors and Mentees

Robert E. Longo, MRC, LPC, BCN
Richard Soutar, PhD, BCN

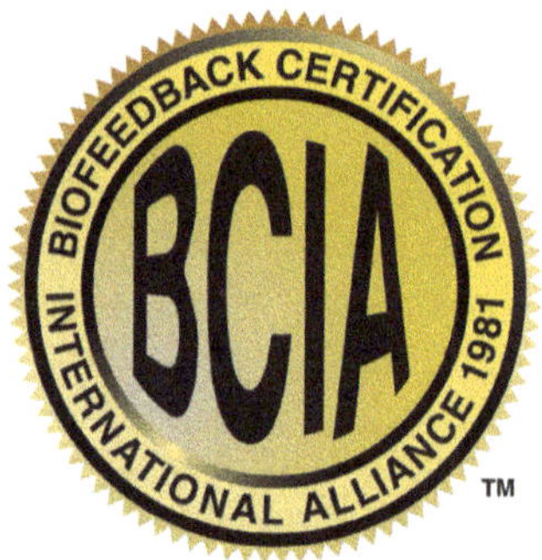

Biomedical

Publisher:
The FNNR
The Foundation for Neurofeedback & Neuromodulation Research
2131 Woodruff Rd, Ste 2100 #121
Greenville, SC 29607
http://www.theFNNR.org
Correspondence: admin@theFNNR.org

Publisher:
The FNNR
The Foundation for Neurofeedback & Neuromodulation Research
2131 Woodruff Rd, Ste 2100 #121
Greenville, SC 29607
http://www.theFNNR.org
Correspondence: Admin@theFNNR.org

Becoming Certified in Neurofeedback: A Guide to the Neurofeedback Mentoring Process for Mentors and Mentees
ISBN: 978-0-9978194-5-8
Layout Design and Cover Graphics: Megan Stevens
Correspondence: Publishing@theFNNR.org

Endorsements

Richard Soutar, PhD, and Rob Longo, MRC are highly respected in the fields of Neurofeedback and Biofeedback. Richard was previously the President of AAPB. They are not salesmen. They do not use puffery, sensationalism, or bells and whistles to try to sell a product. They are truly honest and decent persons, and superb teachers and clinicians. Richard is one of the most astute and knowledgeable, yet approachable, individuals you will encounter in the field of Neurofeedback. He will give you the least-biased, fairest assessment of the state of neurofeedback today..

- John Hummer, PhD, BCN

Contents

Introduction

We have been mentoring professionals in Neurofeedback for many years. In the process leading to BCIA Board Certification in Neurofeedback, we have both taught professionals how to do neurofeedback as well as learned from them the ways to best teach and the typical obstacles they face as beginners in this field. Additionally, we have come to understand the challenges that face even seasoned neurofeedback providers.

Given our years of mentoring experiences, we have repeatedly found that mentees have common challenges, questions, and obstacles that they face and need to work through. When you first start out in Neurofeedback, you are going to feel lost for a while. This is completely normal. Once you grasp the basic concepts, you will then learn at deeper and deeper levels. It is our intent with this manual to address those issues as well inform the reader of the information they need to maximize the mentoring experience.

Additionally, seasoned neurofeedback providers who decide to pursue certification often face challenges when changing equipment, learning new methods, and addressing different disorders.

While there are several certification bodies available to the practitioner, for purposes of this manual we are guiding the reader to prepare for certification by BCIA which is, to the best of our knowledge, the most widely used and well-respected organization providing certification to neurofeedback practitioners that is based on the current science and not tied to one person's theory or the products they sell.

The world of neuroscience is continuously expanding and this in turn results in new knowledge and developments in the field of neurofeedback. As the field matures and advances, BCIA updates its requirements for Certification. Today, the requirements to earn a Board Certification in Neurofeedback (BCN) have changed from a decade ago.

BCIA made its most recent changes and updates at the time we began to write this manual. We have included much of the materials you will find on the BCIA website to facilitate ease of learning and use of information.

We have also found that the process of mentoring is a learning experience. We find that over time we develop improved ways to mentor others and we learn to anticipate the problems and challenges mentees face as well as the challenges put to us as mentors. As mentors we try to build a library of case examples, handouts, and articles to share with those we mentor.

If you are unsure of your intent to pursue your BCN, we believe that the BCIA standards of education and hands-on learning will train you well and will give you the confidence you need to add this exciting modality to your practice.1

Chapter One - What is BCIA[I]?

This section of the manual provides an overview of many of the key elements we believe you need to know if you are being mentored and planning to become BCIA certified in neurofeedback. All text that is italicized is copied from the BCIA website with permission to facilitate the mentoring process.

The Biofeedback Certification International Alliance (BCIA), formerly the Biofeedback Institute of America, was created in 1981 with the primary mission to certify individuals who meet education and training standards in biofeedback and progressively recertify those who advance their knowledge through continuing education. In 1996 the Board of Directors of the Biofeedback Certification Institute of America and the Academy of Certified Neurotherapists collaborated to develop a specialty certification in EEG Biofeedback to be managed and administered by BCIA. The opportunity to certify through the grandparenting process ended on December 31, 1997. Since 1998 the formal certification program in EEG Biofeedback has been available. In March of 2010, BCIA adopted a new name to reflect their global identity and became the Biofeedback Certification International Alliance.

BCIA is an autonomous nonprofit corporation. BCIA policies and procedures are set by an independent board of directors, comprised of a rotating group of distinguished biofeedback clinicians, researchers, and educators.

Board certification is the mark of distinction for providers of biofeedback and neurofeedback services. Certification is valid for 4 years for providers who carry the credential in Biofeedback and Neurofeedback, and 3 years for those who are certified in Pelvic Muscle Dysfunction Biofeedback. Recertification indicates continuous peer review of ethical practice and the acquisition of advanced knowledge of recent developments in the field through required continuing education.

Board certification establishes that an individual has met entry-level requirements for the practice of biofeedback. However, BCIA certification is not a substitute for a state-issued license or other credential to

---

I Reproduced with permission from www.bcia.org

practice one's profession. Candidates for certification who do not hold a professional license, or its equivalent must stipulate that they practice under the supervision of a licensed provider when treating a medical or psychological disorder.

BCIA is recognized as the certification body for the practice of biofeedback by the Association of Applied Psychophysiology and Biofeedback (AAPB), the Biofeedback Federation of Europe (BFE), and the International Society for Neurofeedback and Research (ISNR).

Mission: *BCIA certifies individuals who meet educational and training standards in biofeedback and progressively recertifies those who advance their knowledge through continuing education.*

BCIA endorses the American Psychological Association "Multicultural Guidelines." BCIA professionals recognize the importance of multiculturalism and diversity in clinical and optimal performance practice, education, and research, and treat individuals from diverse ethnic, linguistic, racial, sexual orientation, and gender identity backgrounds with appreciation and sensitivity.

What Does BCIA Certification Entail?

BCIA certificants reported in a comprehensive survey that they initially sought certification for credibility, validation of their skills and knowledge, professional satisfaction, to ensure proper training, and to promote the field. BCIA neurofeedback certification is internationally recognized for six reasons (listed below).

1. BCIA is a non-profit institute that has been an effective advocate for our field. BCIA has been dedicated to a singular mission since 1981:

"BCIA certifies individuals who meet education and training standards in biofeedback and progressively recertifies those who advance their knowledge through continuing education."

2. BCIA's neurofeedback certification is the only program that is recognized by the three major international membership organizations: The Association for Applied Psychophysiology and Biofeedback (AAPB), the Biofeedback Federation of Europe (BFE), and the International Society for Neurofeedback and Research (ISNR).

3. BCIA's neurofeedback certification is based on scientific evidence published in refereed journals. BCIA rejects narrow, unsubstantiated perspectives and the conflict of interest that exists when certification depends on a specific vendor's equipment, databases, and protocols.

BCIA's neurofeedback certification is based on a reading list, Blueprint of Knowledge, and Professional Standards and Ethical Principles that were developed following an extensive job analysis and that are regularly updated by a task force of international authorities in neurofeedback. BCIA continually gathers data to validate and revise its exams through the psychometric process to ensure the relevance, integrity, and value of our certification program.

4. BCIA's neurofeedback certification exam adheres to the highest psychometric standards. We painstakingly evaluate and revise our exam on a regular basis. Several independent experts, who include clinicians and the most experienced educators in our field, regularly review exam items to ensure that the they represent key blueprint concepts, are sourced to our suggested reading list, and are psychometrically sound. We regularly replace outdated exam questions with new ones that are contributed by neurofeedback authorities and then validated by our certificants.

5. BCIA requires that our certificants adhere to one of the strongest ethical codes in our field. In addition, we require that our certificants complete 3 hours of ethics continuing education when they renew their certification. Our rigorous ethical standards are one of the many reasons that our international colleagues have chosen BCIA neurofeedback certification.

6. BCIA's Board of Directors consists of clinicians, educators, and researchers who have guided the development of neurofeedback. Our Board includes leaders of the three major international membership organizations who have contributed decades of service to our field.

Types of Certification in Neurofeedback

1. Neurofeedback Certification *Entry-Level Certification (ELC). The practitioner must hold a license in the State in which she/he practices if they wish to use neurofeedback to independently diagnose a disorder. Unlicensed providers may work under the legal supervision of a licensed provider or in peak or optimal performance.*

Entry-Level Certification (ELC) is designed for the professional who can document a minimum of a BA/BS in a BCIA-approved health care field earned at a regionally accredited academic institution and who has less than 5 years of experience using neurofeedback with patients/clients.

Certification by Prior Experience (CPE) is offered to those licensed professionals with more than 5 years-experience providing neurofeedback services and a minimum of 100 hours of accredited, blueprint-relevant course work that includes a 36-hour didactic course.

2. Technician Neurofeedback Certification - *Technician Certification in neurofeedback is only available for those who are employed by an appropriately licensed and BCIA certified professional who is legally able to provide supervision. Certified technicians will not be listed on the BCIA Find a Practitioner area.*

There is a CPE program for Technicians as well that is based on the years of experience and neurofeedback-specific training.

All certification programs include:

- *Neuroanatomy*
- *Didactic training*
- *Mentoring to learn the application of hands-on skills*
- *Written certification exam*

Chapter Two - Mentoring Guidelines

When you decide to pursue BCIA Certification make sure you REGISTER with BCIA!

BCIA has adopted *Mentoring Guidelines* to provide a framework for this process. These guidelines include contact hours to be spent with a mentor to review personal training, case study presentations, and patient/client sessions. Both the mentor and the BCIA candidate should be familiar with these guidelines. In addition to the guidelines below, as a mentee, you are encouraged to use and review with your mentor the *BCIA Essential Skills List* during the process (see Appendix 3), to test your knowledge. A signed copy must be submitted as a requirement of mentoring.

The Biofeedback Certification International Alliance Guidelines & Policies for Mentoring Candidates for Board Certification in Neurofeedback

BCIA believes that mentoring is essential to ensuring quality in the delivery of neurofeedback services and that it is critical to the training of beginning providers. This document is intended to provide a framework for mentoring of candidates for Board Certification. We recognize that each state has its own definitions and regulations of professionals who offer neurofeedback services. Both the mentor and BCIA candidate should operate within applicable local, state, and federal laws as well as in accordance with the ethical principles of their profession/occupation. Mentoring does not substitute for supervision required for professional licensure or supervision required for insurance reimbursement.

Definitions

An individual becomes a BCIA candidate for certification by submitting an application with documentation of the educational prerequisite and payment of a filing fee. Mentoring is the process of transmitting knowledge and skills from the trained to the untrained or the experienced to the inexperienced practitioner. Mentoring also involves a relationship between a mentor and candidate that promotes the development of skill, knowledge, responsibility and ethical standards in the practice of biofeedback. Through mentoring, the candidate learns to apply knowledge to specific practice situations.

Purpose

Mentoring is unique in that it can provide guidance and support that is not available through any other source of professional development. Ideally, mentoring can be a professionally rewarding experience for both mentor and candidate, enhancing the quality of work and ultimately benefit the patient/client and the public.

Mentoring of BCIA Candidates

I. Obligation of the Mentor
Experienced professionals have an obligation to provide mentoring to those entering the field, thus ensuring that new providers are adequately trained.

II. Qualifications
The following criteria are required for an individual to serve as a mentor of a candidate for BCIA certification.

A. BCIA Certification

The mentor must be BCIA certified. Occasionally, because of geographic location or other special circumstances, a candidate cannot be mentored by a professional who is BCIA certified. If there is a professional available who by exceptional merit and experience would be able to provide appropriate mentoring, a special review of his/her credentials is requested prior to starting training.

B. Experience

The mentor must have at least two years experience in the practice of neurofeedback and with a similar anticipated client base as the candidate.

C. Mentor Qualifications and Limitations

1. A mentor should operate within applicable local, state, and federal laws as well as in accordance with the ethical principles of their profession/ occupation. Mentors should operate within the limits of their expertise, training and professional license/credential.
2. Mentorship does not substitute for supervision required for professional licensure or supervision required for insurance reimbursement. These are unique and separate contractual agreements between two professionals.

D. Professional Commitment

BCIA expects mentors to:

1. Be active in the field of neurofeedback and their professional area as evidenced by affiliations with professional organizations and as required for BCIA recertification.
2. Be free of active sanction by a disciplinary proceeding.
3. Demonstrate involvement in formalized training and participation in professional development in the practice of mentoring. This may include workshops, continuing education programs, and study of current literature.
4. Have expertise with the candidate's client population and methods of practice.
5. Be knowledgeable about issues related to diversity such as race, language, culture, gender, sexual orientation, age, and disability.
6. Be both technically and clinically experienced with a major time and career commitment to the field of applied psychophysiology and biofeedback.

E. Client Confidentiality

BCIA encourages clinicians to maintain HIPPA compliant communication methods for all electronic communications. This would include communications with mentors, colleagues, other professionals and insurance companies. Such compliance would include, but not be limited to, use of coded numbers in place of names, using initials, altered birth dates, blacking out identifying information, or other means of making patient identification impossible. BCIA encourages individuals to check *with their employer, risk manager, or the HIPPA regulations to make certain they are in compliance.*

III. Procedures

A. The BCIA certificant should file a Mentor Application and await approval from BCIA prior to beginning training. A new application should be filed for each prospective candidate.

B. BCIA strongly encourages each prospective candidate to file their certification application and have it approved prior to beginning training.

C. BCIA recommends a written agreement for mentoring which should be signed by both the mentor and candidate prior to starting to work together. It should be amended and renegotiated as needed to reflect any necessary changes. The agreement should include but not be limited to the following:

1. *Obligations of the mentor and the candidate.*
2. *A set period of time (no more than one year) or renegotiated at the end of the time.*
3. *A statement to abide by the ethical principles of the mentor's profession and the BCIA Professional Standards and Ethical Principles of Biofeedback.*
4. *A plan to address conflicts between mentor and candidate.*
5. *A fee charged for mentoring.*
6. *A process for termination of mentoring relationship.*
7. *An evaluation or performance appraisal to be done at specified intervals.*
8. *Format and scheduling of conflict-resolution.*

D. Mentoring should be documented by both the mentor and candidate.

E. We strongly advise that the mentor verify the professional liability insurance of the candidate when the treatment of patients is involved.

F. Original signatures for all phases of mentoring should be provided to BCIA.

IV. Liability Issues

Although it is rare for a mentor to be held liable for the mistakes made by a candidate, we advise prudence when the treatment of patients is involved. It is ill advised to treat patients without obtaining professional liability insurance. In order to avoid liability problems, we strongly advise that the following risk management procedures be instituted by the mentor.

A. Monitor the candidate's professional functioning as well as the mentoring process on a regular basis. Document all interactions.

B. Ensure that neurofeedback services are performed according to accepted standards.

C. To protect patient confidentiality, a mentor should insist on an informed consent form regarding disclosure of information if the identity of the client/patient is evident.

D. Identify any practice that might pose a danger to patients/ clients and quickly take remedial action.

E. Identify any inability to practice due to impairment by alcohol, drugs, illness, stress or personal problems.

V. The Mentoring Relationship

Mentors must maintain objectivity and have no conflict of interest. The mentoring relationship is important because it should promote the development of knowledge and skills and standards of care. Although the mentor is in a position of power, the candidate must be treated with respect. This position must not be used to exploit the candidate in any way, including sexual harassment.

The mentor also has an obligation to the patients/clients of the candidate, and must take appropriate action against unethical conduct of the candidate and one's self. If the mentor believes that the candidate is unqualified to deliver biofeedback services, this must be clearly stated through an evaluation or some other appropriate method.

VI. Mentoring Requirements for BCIA Certification

BCIA requires that a mentor application be submitted and approved prior to starting the mentoring process and that a new application be submitted and approved for each prospective candidate.

BCIA recommends that mentoring of neurofeedback training with patients/clients should take place after the candidate is a pre-qualified BCIA applicant and completes didactic training through an accredited training program, unless the training is part of a degree granting program from an accredited college or university that offers course work concurrently with practicum.

All mentoring requirements may be completed through direct contact or through the use of live phone and/or web meetings. Fax and email may be used as supportive technologies to assist in the transfer of information. The only exception is the "direct observation" requirement, which must be met through direct person-to-person observation.

VII. Neurofeedback Mentoring Requirements

The mentoring requirements involve two essential components: practical experience and mentoring contact hours. Mentoring should be provided by a board certified practitioner (BCN) and may be done remotely via e-mail and telephone except for the two hours of required face to face contact.

A. Mentoring Contact Hours

The mentor and candidate must have a minimum of 25 contact hours together. This time is to be used for the review of 10 sessions of personal neurofeedback, 100 patient/client sessions, and 10 case conference presentations. At least two of these hours must involve direct face-to-face observation during which time the mentor is to directly observe the candidate in his/her technical expertise, proficiency in placements of electrodes, patient/client preparation/orientation to neurofeedback procedures, etc. The remaining 23 hours may be accomplished through either face-to-face, electronic, or phone contact or any combination of these means. If distance is prohibitive for this meeting with your mentor, any professional who also meets all the requirements of a BCIA approved mentor may be used to complete the 2 hours of direct observation.

B. Practical experience

***1. Personal Neurofeedback Training**: The mentor should review the candidate's self-regulatory skills demonstrated with no less than 10 sessions (minimum 20 minutes/session) of personal training involving neurofeedback. The candidate may elect to become the patient/client to be taught by the mentor or review their completed neurofeedback sessions with the mentor.*

2. Client Contact: *The mentor should review the candidate's work with patients/clients. Client contact and treatment should be done with a variety of conditions and should involve not less than six clients over a minimum of 10 weeks. This should be done through conducting at least 100 neurofeedback sessions (minimum 20 minutes/session). The mentor should make sure the candidate has good skills in neurofeedback as well as proper and proficient use of equipment and hook-up techniques*

***3. Case Studies:** The candidate should demonstrate good skills in assessment, setting up a treatment plan and treatment sessions. This should be demonstrated with no less than 10 case study presentations. Ideally these should be actual cases being handled by the candidate but it may also involve cases presented by the mentor to broaden the candidate's exposure to a wide variety of cases.*

VIII. Continuing Education Credit

In order to receive accredited (Category A) hours for BCIA recertification, an approved Mentor Application should be on file with BCIA. A mentor may earn 5 Accredited (Category A) hours for each pre-approved candidate who is mentored for a minimum of 15 contact hours.

IX. Mentoring for Non-Credentialed Providers

BCIA has confirmed its support for our BCIA Professional Standards and Ethical Principles of Biofeedback stating that practitioners must operate within applicable local, state, and federal laws as well as in accordance with the ethical principles of their profession/occupation. BCIA requires that when treating a medical or psychological disorder, one must carry a current health care license/credential in a BCIA approved health care field issued by the state in which you practice or agree to work under the supervision of an appropriately credentialed health care professional. Practitioners should also operate within the limits of their expertise, training and professional license. Mentorship does not substitute for supervision required for professional licensure or supervision required for insurance reimbursement.

How to Document Your Hands-on Training

When you have completed the mentoring process including a minimum of 25 hours with review of 10 Cases, 10 personal neurofeedback sessions, and 100 sessions of neurofeedback with patients/clients; your mentor will fill out and complete the section on your application or may use the following form:

Statement of Mentoring for Board Certification in Neurofeedback

I hereby attest that ____ ***name of candidate*** ____ has completed 25 contact hours, including 2 hours of face to face time or internet live observance with me reviewing the following:

5-A____. Personal Neurofeedback Training Demonstrating Ability to Self-Regulate- 10 sessions

5-B____Neurofeedback Treatment with Clients/Patients - 100 sessions: 100 patient/client sessions using neurofeedback or EEG biofeedback.

5-C____ Neurofeedback Case Studies - 10 Presentations

Mentor's Signature: ____________________ Phone: _______________

Print Name: ______________________ BCIA EEG# ________________

Note: *Each mentor should edit this form appropriately to represent the work that was truly done with each client.*

Note: *BCIA now offers mentoring webinars that, upon live participation or reviewing the recording and the completion of the evaluation and exam process, will award 1 contact hour and 2 case conference presentations. Please be sure to pick only those designated as neurofeedback. We recommend that these webinars not be taken all at once at the beginning of your training but rather take place over the full mentoring timeline so that you will gain the most benefit from these presentations. This is a great way to learn from the best and expand your knowledge!*

Chapter Three - Beginning the Mentoring Process

There is no right or wrong way to begin the Neurofeedback (NFB) mentoring process. You and your mentor should discuss and agree to times to meet, fees for mentoring, documentation, and any other related items (see Appendix 1 -Sample Mentoring Contract). Most important, is to understand what counts towards BCIA mentoring hours and what does not. However, many professionals new to the mentoring process and neurofeedback will have many more questions than seasoned practitioners and may need more instruction in particular areas. For example, conducting brain maps and learning how to interpret findings is important to understanding EEG, but such training is not considered as part of the neurofeedback mentoring process. In some cases, manufacturers of equipment may include how to conduct QEEG Brain Maps as part of their free instruction, while others may not.

Remember: Make sure you register with BCIA. If you do not register with BCIA and begin mentoring and the other requirements you must meet, it could lead to some difficulties later.

The very first thing you should do is be familiar with your computer, the software that runs it, i.e., Windows 10, and basic navigation on your computer. We have spent hours with mentees teaching them the basics of just how to locate or save files on their computers! If you are struggling with computer basics, it is important that you take the time to learn your system. Have a friend or family member help you or take a basic course. This is a great example of what is NOT mentoring.

Time spent learning to plug in your equipment and getting it to perform is not mentoring. This is a practicum and you must be able to efficiently use your equipment prior to seeing clients and starting the mentoring process. Many equipment vendors will be happy to offer you some training specific to the use of their equipment. This may be a good question to ask prior to purchase.

Often times mentoring is not done in person; instead the services are provided on line using software that allows screen sharing. If you are being mentored on line; it is also important that you purchase a good quality headset with a built-in microphone, in order to prevent unwanted background noise and negative sound feedback.

One of our mentees suggested; "*Before the process starts, ask yourself and discuss with your mentor, the purpose for being mentored.*" Is your purpose to become BCIA Certified? Is your mentoring for personal enrichment? Both? If you are pursuing BCIA mentoring, make sure your mentors are in agreement with and understand the BCIA requirements; otherwise information for multiple mentors can become confusing. If you are engaging in mentoring for personal enrichment, then make sure to talk with your mentor and provide him or her with a list of topics you would like to discuss and log the time spent for tracking purposes. Not all mentors may be able to provide you with the specifics or details you wish to pursue.

In writing this manual, we asked professionals who have gone through the mentoring process to suggest what would be helpful to them during the mentoring process. Their ideas and recommendations are incorporated throughout the next chapter.

One of the first things we recommend is that you purchase your equipment before you get started. If you have selected a mentor, then he/she may be helpful in guiding you to what system you may need. It is also important to note that many professionals and mentors have biases for and in some cases against various pieces of equipment. This is why establishing your budget is important. One of us had a mentee that was looking to buy a piece of equipment and the initial quote was for over $25,000.00. The quote included computers 2 pieces of equipment and advanced software that is not easy to use. It did not include any equipment needed to do QEEG brain maps.

For the new practitioner, this could be financially difficult to get started. The same manufacturer could have made a quote for around $5,000.00 - $6,000.00 which would have included a very good and basic piece of equipment and all the necessary software and hardware to begin doing QEEG brain maps. If you are new to neurofeedback and have a limited budget, then we recommend you purchase a simple two channel or four channel amplifier. Several companies make these pieces of equipment and several come with software to do QEEG brain maps as well. These units fall into the $4,000 to $6,000 range. We would recommend that you go to one of the regional or national conferences on neurofeedback because in most instances the major vendors of neurofeedback equipment are attending and have booths in the vendor area where you can try out equipment and software.

Most equipment is FDA registered and the major manufacturers have years of experience behind their products. Be wary of Internet ads. Many companies are producing devices and games that are advertised as improving brain function, memory, attention, sleep, etc. Some devises do neurofeedback but use fixed electrodes that may only target 2, 4, or 6 of 19+ 10/20 International sites; and may only train at certain brain wave frequencies, i.e., alpha, theta, or beta. Make sure the equipment you buy is designed to do brainwave training at any of the 10/20 international sites and that you can set what bandwidths you want to train up or down and that the equipment can train at specified frequencies.

Some of the companies/vendors who sell equipment, and how to select quality equipment, are listed on the ISNR website https://www.isnr.org/member-list (see Corporate Members) and the AAPB website: http://www.aapb.org/files/LegitimateDevices.pdf

In some cases, your mentor or the vendor can provide you with screen shots or photos of different pieces of equipment with explanations of what is being seen. Some equipment provides the user with a session review screen that shows a completed session that can be compared for purposes of demonstrating good progress, mediocre progress, and minimal to no progress. Mentees often find this information to be very helpful. I

As noted above, there are multiple mapping systems to choose from and those new to the field often feel confused and/or overwhelmed regarding which system is the right one for them. We would suggest to the reader that there are generally two types of mapping systems; those that are detailed and used for research purposes, and those which are more basic and clinically oriented. As a professional you should explore the various systems (many of the manufacturers/ vendors are willing to give perspective clients free trial periods or maps to run so the perspective buyer has the opportunity to test and see that system).

Those new to the field may wish to consider attending one of the national conferences as offered by AAPB and ISNR. The AAPB meeting is in the spring and the ISNR meeting is in the fall. Most of the large vendors are there for you to meet them in person and try out the equipment you may be considering.

It is well worth your time up front to look at these systems and see which one is best for you. Your mentor will often be able to make recommendations. This would also provide you with the opportunity to see a variety of brain mapping systems. Why are we talking about brain mapping since that is not included in our mentoring? Because, many of the professionals who have elected to add neurofeedback to their practice are also aware of QEEG Brain Mapping and often look for systems that do both neurofeedback and QEEG. Some of these systems provide the user with an opportunity to do pre-post comparisons of maps when the client/patient has been mapped before, during and/or after brainwave training is complete. Again, do your homework and compare prices, software options and equipment capabilities BEFORE you invest your money into a system.

If you decide to proceed with doing QEEG brain maps, ask the manufacturer or your mentor about resources that will help you such as the effects of drugs and medications on EEG, common artifact, and other issues that can interfere with getting quality QEEG such as electrical interference.

There are several paradigms in neurofeedback and each is tied to different types of equipment. Many clinical methods and protocols can only be performed on specifically designed pieces of equipment. The software and techniques used can require years of experience with these different softwares and techniques. Most mentors are only familiar with a few paradigms and their associated equipment and software. Consequently, it is important to be sure that your mentor is familiar enough with your system and associated paradigm to be able to guide you expertly. A mentor may be experienced with several qEEG based neurofeedback systems such as Neuroguide, BrainMaster or New Mind but not familiar with the equipment and software you purchased as well as the workshops you attended to do Infra Slow neurofeedback. This can be the same case for LENS, Neurofield, or bipolar training methods used by Sebern Fisher. Even the difference between basic EEGer software and Bioexplorer software can confound efforts to mentor clinicians.

Clinical decisions involving protocol interventions can be limited or expanded by the software and equipment available. A mentor may know how to help your client but your equipment may not be able to implement the protocol he or she knows would be best for the client based on prior experience. This is an unfortunate aspect of a field that is very complex and rapidly developing. You best defense is to be sure you are interested in the paradigm your mentor teaches and that you have the equipment that he or she is familiar enough with to guide you at an optimal level.

Some equipment for neurofeedback also includes the software and ability to conduct other interventions in biofeedback. If you are interested in learning about and providing these services such as heart rate variability (HRV), skin temperature monitoring (Thermofeedback), muscle tension (EMG), photic or audio-visual entrainment (AVE), etc., talk to the manufacturer / vendor of the equipment to learn more about optional features.

Documentation of The Mentoring Process

If you are working with multiple mentors, make sure your mentor and you are documenting each session including date, amount of time, and topics discussed. In fact, it would be a good idea for your mentors to communicate with each other as to what has been covered, areas needing improvement, etc.

Your mentor(s) should also be periodically reviewing with you what mentoring objectives are left and how they will be accomplished in the mentoring process with you. The mentor should track the objective work used to demonstrate progress, and completion of BCIA requirements on a log sheet that can be given to the next mentor if one is being used (See Appendix 4 - BCIA Mentoring Documentation Log). The finished log sheet should satisfy the BCIA requirements in a clear way so that there is no question as to completion and the work (cases used) can be recalled.

If you are just beginning and need to learn the basic such as the 10-20 International System of electrode placement, get yourself a foam head from a beauty supply shop. They cost about $8-10. Type up the various 10-20 sites on a Word document, print them out, and cut out each label.

10 / 20 System Electrode Distances

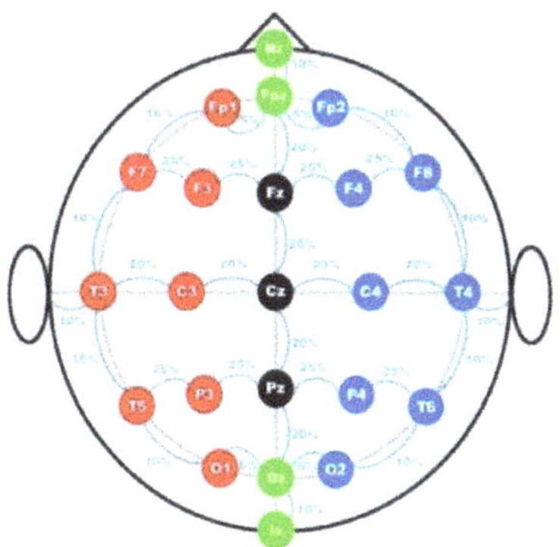

Figure 3. Using the 10-20 model paste or tape them to the foam head in their approximate positions[II]. It will help you learn 10-20 placement more quickly if you can visualize it repeatedly, in 3D. Left hemisphere sites are odd-numbered and right hemisphere sites are evenly numbered. You start off a map with site Fp1 and go sequentially first around the 'hat band' area: Fp1, F7, T3, T5, O1, Oz, O2, T6, T4, F8, Fp2, and Fpz. Next, you go around the 'beanie' or 'yarmulke' area: F3, C3, P3, Pz, P4, C4, and F4. Lastly, the midline: Fz, and Cz. Montages get a bit confusing. The standard monopolar montage is ground on one ear (usually left), reference on right ear, and active on the scalp. Resist the feeling of insecurity and urge to buy lots of different equipment. A two-channel or four-channel is all that you need. You want a company with good technical support. Try to find equipment which is very intuitive and user friendly, with a lot of point and click, and menus, to make things very easy.

II (e.g. http://www.ers-education.org/lrmedia/2016/pdf/298830.pdf)

Chapter Four - The Mentoring Process

BCIA Certification Requirements – Neurofeedback Mentoring

This section will focus on learning the hands-on skills, called the mentoring process, and recommendations to help your mentoring process go more smoothly and efficiently. The process of mentoring involves a relationship between a mentor and candidate that promotes the development of skills, knowledge, responsibility, and ethical standards in the practice of neurofeedback. Neurofeedback practitioners cross a variety of health-related disciplines including Counseling, Social Work, Psychology, Medicine, Chiropractic, Nursing, Nurse Practitioners, Physical Therapy, among many other disciplines.

While there are a variety of mentors who are BCIA approved mentors, not every mentee will be able to select a mentor who is both BCIA Certified and approved as well as a licensed practitioner in the same field or discipline. This should not create a problem for the mentee because BCIA Mentors are not providing clinical supervision. Mentors are providing guidance and education in the application of neurofeedback services. Clinical supervision is provided by a licensed practitioner who is legally able to take responsibility for another person's work. This is regulated by state licensing boards specific to each profession and may differ between states. If you are considering working under supervision, please check with this intended supervisor to be sure they have read and carefully considered their practice standard guidelines.

To become a BCIA approved mentor, mentors are required to meet two qualifications:

1. *The mentor must have a current, valid BCIA certification.*
2. *The mentor must have two years of experience using neurofeedback as a significant portion of his/her work.*

There is an application to be filed with BCIA and upon approval, it will be valid for one year. During that time, one can add new mentees to the list. If there has been a major change in your practice or professional status, BCIA asks to be notified immediately as it could have an impact on the status of providing mentoring services.

Because most mentors do charge a fee, BCIA takes this very seriously and BCIA wants you (the mentee), to learn more about how to find the right person who is a good match for your skill set and your interests. For example, if your client-base is largely children diagnosed with ADHD, your mentor should also have good experience with this population.

Having more than one mentor is not only permissible, but in some cases advisable. The most important thing to remember is to log your contact time and what was accomplished after each session. Many people find this log sheet to be helpful (see Appendix 4). This sheet is for your use and does not need to be submitted to BCIA for certification. When tracking time with the mentor, be sure to track contact time and what was accomplished. Was it reviewing your personal neurofeedback session or was it the review of time you spent with a specific client.

Do Not Be Confused

BCIA mentoring is a specialized relationship with specific aspects as to what must be done to complete the process; and what constitutes mentoring activities and what does not. First and foremost, mentoring is just that. It is a professional relationship in which the mentor (an experienced person) trains, guides, and assists the mentee (an inexperienced or less experienced person) in acquiring and developing a specific set of skills and knowledge that will expand and enhance the mentee's professional knowledge and skills.

Mentoring is NOT supervision. Clinical supervision is generally performed by a licensed professional who is approved by a state board and must follow specific guidelines as defined by the state licensing board for purposes of a supervisee acquiring licensure in their specific area of study or degree, (i.e., counseling, social work, psychology). Additionally, supervision can also mean a licensed professional takes legal responsibility for the work of an unlicensed person. This is defined and regulated by state law and is not specific to neurofeedback. This is very important to know the distinctions because some mentees may continue to call you from time to time for advice; however, you are NOT their supervisor unless you have made a formal and legal arrangement.

As noted above BCIA mentoring has specific requirements to be met: 10 Case Studies, 10 personal neurofeedback sessions and 100 client patient sessions to be reviewed by the mentor(s). Thus, conducting a QEEG Brain Map is NOT required, and conducting a brain map and QEEG interpretation do not count towards BCIA certification however, a QEEG may be used as part of a case study.

Operating a computer, installation and operation of software, equipment functions and use do not count as credit towards BCIA certification. In fact, BCIA encourages the mentee to already have basic training and experience in these areas BEFORE starting the mentoring process.

While BCIA required case studies may include difficult cases, case consultation outside of addressing neurofeedback specific concerns, may need to occur in addition to a BCIA case study review with your mentor(s); and may require consulting with a clinical supervisor. Case consultation in and of itself is not required as part of the BCIA mentoring process. This would fall more-so under the definition of a clinical consult or part of clinical supervision. For example, many seasoned professionals in our field will send an odd map out for comment or will have a client that is not responding as expected. They call another professional or even post a note on a list serv. This is not mentoring - just asking for outside input or case consultation.

Both Sides

We decided to write this book for both ***Mentor*** and ***Mentee*** so both persons involved understand the mentoring process from both sides. Therefore, as you read this book, it will address core issues from the perspective of both parties. For example: ***Case Studies***

A case study refers to all of the neurofeedback work done with a client from intake and protocol selection/adjustment, through treatment and on to discharge.

Mentor: The mentee needs a total of 10 case studies. The goal of this type of learning is to expose the mentee to additional scenarios and more clients. The mentee can present all 10 if they have not been previously discussed with your mentor nor included as part of the 100 sessions. As a mentor you can also provide case studies. You may wish to look at the experience of your mentee and pick a few of your cases that you believe would illustrate something important and fill in any learning gaps. This is a good way to use group mentoring as it can save your time and can save money for the mentees. You pick a case and tell it to many students together and they can all learn, ask questions, and get credit for the session. BCIA Webinars have several case study presentations which the mentee may view and acquire credit for towards their mentoring requirements.

Mentee: You must have a total of 10 case studies. If you do not have a large client/patient case load, you may get credit from your mentor presenting case studies to you, or you may attend, or review webinars conducted by BCIA to get case study credits.

In this section we will go over a variety of basic concepts and requirements related to the mentoring process.

QEEG Brain Maps

NOTE: Learning the process of conducting a QEEG Brain Map, editing raw EEG, and reviewing QEEG results is not a part of the BCIA Neurofeedback mentoring process.

The field of neurofeedback practitioners do not all agree that using QEEG Brain Maps is essential and/or important. However, a growing number of practitioners do use QEEG, and these practitioners believe it is essential in order to provide more accurate and high-quality neurofeedback. For those interested in learning highly specialized forms of Neurofeedback, i.e., sLORETA, Z-Score Training; QEEG-guided neurofeedback provides you with optimum guidance in protocol selection, electrode placement, and outside of self-report, the best measure of neurofeedback efficacy with a particular patient when remapped.

QEEG informs the choice of training sites, but there are various informed strategies that one might use. For example, nuanced adjustments to reinforcement rates on the fly in order to elicit the client's best performance. This is applied science at its best – a collaborative, flexible approach where the client is educated in how they can change the functioning and structure of their own brain, through a nonlinear dynamic process.

Some clinicians may tell you that you should have all your QEEG raw data reviewed by a qualified professional, i.e., a Neurologist. This is simply not true. There are several QEEG mapping systems that take raw data and convert the data into a brain map. In some cases, if you observe unusual brain wave activity when acquiring a map, then having the raw data reviewed by a qualified professional would be in order; however, unless you have had some basic training in QEEG acquisition and interpretation, then you would not likely know what constitutes problematic EEG. But for purposes of being mentored, again, conducting QEEGs is not a part of or required to become BCIA certified.

This differs from a one size fits all approach of plug and play neurofeedback when the uninformed practitioner is relying upon technology alone, without understanding the interplay of brain functioning and focused states of attention (facilitated by immediate feedback of one's performance) or concepts such as compensatory processes and stages of reorganization.

Mentor: It is not our job to promote nor sell any particular brand of equipment. It is best to provide the mentee with a list of manufacturers/vendors of which you are familiar as well as a list of brain mapping systems from which the mentee can select; again, and ones with which you are familiar.

Mentee: There are a variety of manufactures and vendors of neurofeedback equipment available from prices as low as $6,000 up to $30,000. Some Neurofeedback equipment/systems are capable of conducting QEEG brain maps and others are not. There are also a variety of QEEG Brain Map systems and software you can chose from and most work with the various types of equipment. Your mentor should be able to discuss with you the pros and cons of each system and software without bias.

Scope of Practice

A mentee's scope of practice is one of the most important considerations in the BCIA mentoring process. If you are applying for ***Technician Neurofeedback Certification,*** this means you do not have a license to practice in your state and thus your scope of practice is limited to the cases for which you are being supervised (i.e., you should not be treating medical disorders if you are not being supervised by a medical professional). BCIA certified technicians must be supervised by a Licensed and BCIA Certified practitioner who is able to provide supervision of your neurofeedback sessions. Neurofeedback technicians must work in accordance with the practice standard guidelines of the supervising licensed practitioner. Therefore, if your supervising practitioner focuses on peak performance with neurofeedback, then self-regulation skills would be the focus of your client caseload. As a technician working for a peak performance trainer, you cannot claim to be treating any medical, mental health, or diagnosable disorders.

If you are applying for ***Neurofeedback Certification***, then you may only claim to treat the disorders covered in your scope of practice. For example, as a masters level counselor, you can train clients for improved relaxation and self-regulation skills. You can treat mental health disorders such as anxiety and depression; however, you cannot claim to treat medical disorders such as migraine, ADHD, insomnia, etc. To do so would be practicing outside of your scope of practice.

If you are mentoring a licensed counselor teaching client's relaxation and self-regulation skills to help with stress headaches, then you would be within your scope of practice. So, what do you do if you get a referral for a medical disorder? If a medical doctor refers a patient to you to treat a medical disorder; how should you proceed? You might talk with the doctor about what the etiology of the disorder. If the diagnosis is insomnia, you can treat a client/patient for self-regulation and relaxation skills which in turn helps the patient relax, remain calm and better manage their stress.

Selecting a Mentor

Locating a mentor who is a good match for your career goals is very important. You may use more than one mentor, however, you and all of your mentors you should keep accurate records, to ensure that you are logging the experience in terms of contact hours and the activity reviewed: personal training sessions, patient/client sessions, and case studies. Appendix 3 is the BCIA form used to document mentoring sessions. The form is designed to serve as a guide to help you track your progress and does not need to be submitted. Each mentor is required to sign off on mentoring requirements they personally completed.

Keep in mind; Dual relationships – The APA is quite clear about dual relationships and in accordance with their guidelines, one should not provide BCIA mentoring for a family member. As for supervision, this is an issue handled by the appropriate licensing board. Remember, BCIA Mentoring is NOT supervision.

Mentor: You should provide a copy of this form for your mentee to keep record of and track requirements for each mentoring session.

Mentee: Make sure you have a copy of this form, so you can keep a personal record of dates and times of your mentoring sessions and topics/requirements covered during each session.

Mentoring may be done using various distance methods where you communicate and review training sessions electronically. Remember if you are unlicensed and do not have access to equipment and clients, you may find mentoring to be a more difficult process. In fact, you may be looking for an internship. This is important to know before you start to research mentors. You will be truly asking a BCN mentor to use their equipment and their clients. Be prepared to ask a prospective mentor specifically what you need.

We also encourage you to select a mentor who is familiar with the type of equipment you purchase, as well as the type of neurofeedback methods you are practicing; i.e., traditional 1, 2 and 4 channel neurofeedback; Z-Score training; full cap training; sLORETA training, ISL, etc.

We recommend you begin your mentoring with learning about traditional neurofeedback. This will provide you with a strong foundation to build upon when learning other techniques. The bulk of research in using neurofeedback to treat various conditions and disorders has been done using traditional neurofeedback methods and protocols.

Mentoring is absolutely necessary to learn proper technique, basics of map interpretation, and to make sense of what is happening during a training session. Few books will provide you with the depth of information you need to practice effective neurofeedback.

When your mentor incorporates cutting edge information from research and practice, in order for you to grasp concepts such as compensation, plasticity, signal to noise ratio, and inter-hemispheric communication, you gain a better in-depth understanding of the field.

Books, Articles, and Resources

There are good strategies that give the practitioner an edge in providing neurofeedback services. In addition to recommended books and readings (listed in Appendix 5); compiling a library of resources, including video-recorded special topics presentations by experts in various holistic fields related to neurofeedback; participating in an interactive online list-serve; individual mentoring sessions; conferences and workshops; and webinars are various methods you can use to advance your knowledge, skills, and abilities.

Neurofeedback can be frustrating, but if one can manage the initial frustration and confusion, lasting benefits will be reaped for the practitioner and the clients they serve. It is an ongoing learning process, always exciting and challenging. And it is truly collaborative and scientific, with you, the informed guide, helping the motivated client undergo a process of growth and transformation.

Mentor: You should be prepared to provide mentees with titles of books, articles, and print resources to help them learn about Neurofeedback. In addition, you should encourage membership in organizations that are focused on Neurofeedback as well as joining listserves of these organizations, i.e., AAPB, ISNR, and the various state and regional societies specific to the field. Additionally, sharing books and articles and/or directing the mentee to resources where he or she can acquire articles on various neurofeedback related topics is always helpful.

Mentee: Ask your mentor about organizations to join that are focused on neurofeedback. A list of core readings is listed in Appendix 5; and a list of recommended readings is supplied in Appendix 6. Your mentor should be able to steer you to places where you can find articles, papers, etc., on neurofeedback. In addition, organizations such as AAPB, ISNR, BCIA, and state/regional societies offer webinars on various related topics. Many vendors, manufacturers, and practitioners offer webinars on a variety of neurofeedback related topics.

Topics to Cover During Mentoring

While BCIA requires you to have 10 case studies, have 10 neurofeedback sessions on yourself to review with your mentor, and review 100 client/patient neurofeedback sessions with you mentor, there is also an Essential Skills List (see Appendix 3) that you will need to review and have signed off by with your mentor. Some of those topics are listed but not inclusive of the list of topics that follow.

Client/Patient Orientation

When providing neurofeedback, the practitioner and/or technician should be able explain to a new client, in layman's terms and simple language:

- What is neurofeedback,
- Self-regulation concepts,
- Operant conditioning of brainwave activity,
- The major stages in the neurofeedback treatment/training

process, from initial intake and assessment to progress monitoring and reporting.

In addition, the patient/client should understand his/her role and responsibilities in the neurofeedback process (see sample form Appendix 8). At the initial session, the practitioner and/or technician should be able to explain how the neurofeedback session process and equipment works, including:

- The purpose and steps involved in skin preparation,
- The steps in electrode attachment and selection of site placements; and to assure client/patient about safety of "sensors"/electrodes,
- The meaning of primary features of the feedback screens and concepts of amplitude and frequency and/or z-scores,
- The relationship between client activity and on-screen feedback changes, and
- The session recording and progress monitoring screens.

Finally, the practitioner and/or technician should obtain written client/patient permission for treatment/ training using a thorough Informed Consent form (see Appendix 7).

Mentors: Use the Essential Skills list to assure the mentee can explain/ demonstrate the associated skills.

Mentees: Use the Essential Skills checklist with your mentor(s) as a guide to assure you are engaging in the minimal activities for proper client/patient orientation.

Intake, Assessment and Protocol Selection

In a neurofeedback practice, regardless of the practitioner's/ technician's background, training, and experience; it is important to be able to demonstrate and document a thorough client symptom and medication history and gather background information relevant to treatment/training goals.

Whether or not you are using QEEG Brain Mapping, the practitioner and/or technician should be able to provide a thorough EEG baseline assessment, using the following skills

- Perform correct measurements to name and locate on the scalp each of the International 10-20 System electrode placement sites,
- Properly prepare scalp and ears and attach electrodes to selected assessment sites, or, attach an electrode cap if doing a full-cap quantitative EEG,
- Correctly perform all steps to collect a QEEG recording or multi-channel EEG assessment: checking impedances, removing artifact, and collecting eyes-open and eyes-closed data,
- Demonstrate basic understanding of a QEEG assessment report, as well as the most commonly reported components of QEEG databases (absolute power, relative power, phase, coherence, z-score comparisons, etc.),
- Identify recordings indicating spike and wave activity requiring consultation with a neurologist or QEEG expert,
- Use all intake, psychometric, and baseline EEG data to select target electrode placement sites and montages for neurofeedback treatment/training, and
- Select an initial neurofeedback protocol and explain rationale to client

Mentees: If you are not doing QEEGs on your patients/clients, your mentor should be able to assist you in how to determine protocol selection and the best methods of monitoring client/patient progress from reviewing EEG recordings from neurofeedback sessions.

Mentors: You should be able to clearly and accurately guide the mentee on protocol selection to best address symptoms when QEEG is not used.

Equipment and Types of Neurofeedback

In our opinion, it may be advantageous to have your own equipment before you begin the mentoring process. There are a number of vendors who sell a variety of neurofeedback devices. Take the time to shop and talk to others about various pieces you are interested in. The cost of equipment can also vary greatly. If you are on a tight budget, you might be able to find used equipment for a reasonable price. Vendors may have used/refurbished equipment which you may find financially attractive in the beginning. You might also check with vendors to see if they rent/lease equipment.

Additionally, there are various types of Neurofeedback: traditional, Z-Score, Infra Slow, LENS, and sLORETA, among others. Not all equipment provides the software/options to do all of these methods and some manufacturers charge a fee to have a license for each one. From a practical standpoint, you want to make sure whatever equipment you purchase can do traditional neurofeedback so that you start by learning the basics from the ground up.

But one thing is absolutely certain; at this point in time, there is no compelling evidence that any one approach is superior to any other approach. One needs to be diligent in looking at the published research about neurofeedback efficacy and outcomes; as well as methods that are promoted as being more effective than traditional neurofeedback methods. Research articles should be published in peer reviewed journals. Be leery of self-published papers that may make unrealistic claims. Comparative studies have neither been done, nor replicated. Resist any hype or claims to the contrary. Effectiveness also has a lot to do with the skill and expertise of the practitioner.

We also suggest you select a mentor who is familiar with the equipment you have purchased or plan to purchase. This is important because your mentor should be able to help you set up neurofeedback protocols; work with the software you are using, read the QEEG Maps it generates, troubleshoot hardware and/or software problems, etc.

In as much as there is different equipment to choose from, there are also different QEEG Brain Mapping systems to choose from. Some are better for research endeavors, while others are more clinically focused. The various map generating systems also differ in the type of reports they generate. Many of these companies will offer you a free trial to test their services before you purchase a contract with them.

Use and Maintenance of Neurofeedback Equipment

Unlike many other health related fields, Neurofeedback requires the use of computers, electronic devices, various types of software, and the knowledge to use them efficiently and effectively. And because electronics and software are not flawless and prone to have occasional problems, the practitioner/technician should be very well trained and familiar with the computers, devices and related software they are using. In the world of bicycle racing, they say it is not a matter of IF you will crash, it is a matter of when. In the world of neurofeedback, it is not a matter of if you will have equipment breakdowns, software problems etc., but when you will have them. Often it happens at the beginning or during a neurofeedback session. The technical support provided by vendors is important in this regard. Ask about technical support including response time and costs BEFORE purchasing your equipment.

We have seen practitioners and technicians who have run neurofeedback sessions on a client/ patient without plugging in equipment, using bad electrodes, excessive artifact, etc., without knowing or understanding what they were seeing on the screen. Some practitioners/ technicians set the patient up for a session, start the session and leave the room, and thus not monitoring the quality or efficacy of the session.

The practitioner/technician should be able to demonstrate thorough knowledge of operation of neurofeedback equipment of choice, how to:

- Make correct hardware connections and start hardware,
- Make correct electrode connections to the hardware,
- Identify and remove (or control for) sources of common artifacts in the raw EEG signal,
- Troubleshoot common equipment failures according to manufacturer's recommendations

Additionally, the practitioner/technician should be able to demostrate thorough knowledge of appropriate software for selected equipment by:

- Accurately selecting, installing, and running neurofeedback treatment/training software, and
- Identifying components, applications, and limitations of selected software package.

Mentors: You should be familiar with the equipment the mentee is using to be able to guide, troubleshoot, and resolve common problems the mentee is having learning how to use his/her equiment and software.

Mentees: Make sure the mentor you work with is familiar with the equipment, software, and use of protocols with the equipment you have purchased and are using.

NOTE: *There is a difference between mentoring and equipment practicum -Mentoring can begin when the mentee can demonstrate some basic competence with equipment and is only the time spent reviewing the actual work as outlined by BCIA. Primarily working on equipment issues or technical support is not mentoring and should not be included.*

Neurofeedback Session Management and Reporting

Running neurofeedback sessions is the foundation of using neurofeedback in any given practice. This is why we mentor those new to the field and why being mentored is so important to having a successful neurofeedback practice.

Conducting neurofeedback treatment/training sessions involves the following procedures:

- Provide initial orientation and instructions to clients/patients at the first treatment/training session.
- Review and signing of informed consent, HIPAA, patient's rights and other documents.

- Prior to subsequent sessions, query client (and/or parent) verbally and/or via pre-session questionnaire on client's positive and negative reactions to previous session.
- Maintain basic hygiene procedures in attaching (and cleaning) electrodes, (see Hagedorn, D. 2014[III]).
- Remind client of the training objectives for each session and their role in attending to and responding to feedback.
- Start treatment/training software program, set up selected protocol parameters, and run basic feedback functions.
- As appropriate, set initial training thresholds and adjust as needed.
- Identify and remove sources of artifact appearing in session recordings.
- Monitor session recordings and provide coaching and supplemental verbal feedback to client during sessions, as appropriate.
- Save session data per equipment guidelines and review session results with client.
- Assign homework to client that supports and supplements session training goals.
- Consult with client's prescribing physician and/or providers of other concurrent treatments as necessary to avoid treatment complications and maximize treatment outcomes.
- Identify as soon as possible in the treatment/training process when neurofeedback is not working for a client; identify cause(s) for lack of progress; make necessary protocol or other training program adjustments; or, when necessary, recommend termination of neurofeedback.
- In collaboration with the client, determine when neurofeedback treatment/training goals have been met and mutually plan for treatment termination and follow-up.
- Conduct all aspects of neurofeedback treatment and training in accordance with BCIA, AAPB, and ISNR codes of ethical practice (see The BCIA Professional Standards and Ethical Principles of Biofeedback [PSEP] - Appendix 2).

III Hagedorn, D. (2014). Infection Risk Mitigation for Biofeedback Providers. Biofeedback: Volume 42, Issue 3, pp. 93–95

Mentors: Encourage all mentees to read, understand, and follow the above items, and when appropriate or helpful, share forms you use in your practice if feasible.

Mentees: There are several forms one can use to advise patients/clients of the neurofeedback process, what it entails, and some of the risks/benefits/and challenges in participating in neurofeedback (see Appendices 7, 8, and 9).

In addition, it is important to maintain orderly and up-to-date client files, including, 1) session-by-session training records, significant session events and client comments, 2) changes in client medication, significant life changes, allergies, etc., that may impact treatment/training results, and 3) reports of consultations with other treatment providers, family members, teachers, etc. Appendix 13 is a sample session notation form.

Use of Supplemental Therapeutic and Training Modalities

In addition to the above, BCIA suggests the following items be addressed during the mentoring process when applicable:

1. Demonstrate ability to establish positive, constructive relationships with clients and their family members, using basic counseling/communication skills.
2. Document adequate training and demonstrate skills required to use appropriate counseling /therapy methods to supplement neurofeedback with clients having mental health diagnoses, if applicable.
3. Document adequate training in use of alpha-theta neurofeedback protocols. Demonstrate ability to select appropriate clients for alpha-theta specific neurofeedback protocols training as well as apply appropriate therapy methods when using these protocols.
4. Document adequate training understanding of in other neuromodulation modalities (such as HRV biofeedback, AVS, CES, etc.) for use in conjunction with neurofeedback, and demonstrate ability to select and use appropriate adjunctive modalities with individual clients, if applicable.

These additional modalities may require separate training, equipment, and/or licensure. For example, if one is not trained and licensed in counseling/psychotherapy, then one should not be practicing that form of mental health interventions. If your equipment is not designed to do Alpha Theta neurofeedback training, and if you have not been properly trained/instructed on the use of Alpha Theta training and its risks, then we would recommend you not do this training. Similarly, with other forms of biofeedback like HRV or diaphragmatic breathing, you should get training in these interventions. Use of additional devices and equipment such as AVE or CES require training and, depending upon the manufacturer, may require licensure to acquire the device.

Client/Patient Consults

In our experience, unless the potential patient/client has prior knowledge of neurofeedback training, and understands the basic principles involved with this intervention, offering potential patients the opportunity to come in for a consult prior to being mapped and/or beginning neurofeedback, is strongly encouraged. Potential patients/clients do not always get the most important and, in many cases, the most accurate information from just doing an Internet search. Often the Internet offers varied, and in some case conflicting information. This is a nice opportunity to discuss the fact that you have been properly trained and are working on, or have been Board Certified by BCIA. If supervised, explain to your clients/patients that you are under supervision and by whom.

It is important to keep in mind that potential clients/patient often have common questions that they ask during a consult. How often do I need to have sessions? How long do sessions last? What should I do in-between sessions? How many sessions do I need? What is the cost per session? What if I get sick and miss a session? Do I continue to take my medications? These are just a few of the questions prospective clients/patients might ask.

They may not understand the risks and benefits of neurofeedback training nor the types of disorders that may benefit from such.

In our experience the overwhelming majority of patients/clients who come in for an initial consult will agree to have a QEEG done (if offered) and of those who have a QEEG, over 95% will agree to sign on for neurofeedback training. Therefore, risks and benefits should be addressed during the initial consult.

Mentors: This is an excellent opportunity to help the mentee address some of the concepts already discussed above. Initial client/patient – Practitioner contact is what helps build a good neurofeedback practice.

Mentees: Your mentor should be able to instruct you in various methods, concepts, and ideas for having initial patient/client consults. Your mentor may share basic forms that clients/patients need to sign (examples are in the Appendices), should the person decide to engage in neurofeedback training.

Print Information for Clients/Patients

Some of the forms many clinics, practices and programs using neurofeedback use include; Informed Consent (see Appendix 7), Client Bill of Rights and Responsibilities (see Appendix 8), QEEG Brain Mapping Preparation Checklist (see Appendix 12), Client Acknowledgements (see Appendix 9), Authorization for Release of Information - HIPAA (see Appendix 10) Financial Policy (see Appendix 11).

These forms are useful, and in some cases necessary, to meet the ethical standards and practices of neurofeedback practitioners and technicians. They provide both you and the patient/client with a layer of protection and safety.

In addition, many clinics and practitioners create information sheets/ brochures that provide the potential patient/client with basic information about neurofeedback and QEEG[IV]. These can be left in a waiting room for patients/clients as well as distributed to referral sources.

IV See: Longo, R.E. (2018) A Consumer's Guide to Understanding QEEG Brain Mapping and Neurofeedback Training.

Interpretation of Neurofeedback Sessions/Trend Screens from Session to Session

This is one of the major requirements toward becoming efficient and effective in providing neurofeedback services and a major requirement of the BCIA Certification process. This is not something you will learn from reading a book and requires guidance by an experienced practitioner.

Progress determination will be based upon the post-session data collected from your sessions. Whether you are using traditional neurofeedback; 1, 2, and/or 4 Channel training; or specialized neurofeedback methods such as LENS, Z-score, sLORETA, Infra-Slow, Infra-Low, etc., it is important to be able to understand and describe what occurred during any neurofeedback session. Were there integration, magnitude or coherence changes? Were targeted areas affected? What was the overall training efficiency? These and other areas of change pre-post session are critical to becoming efficient in providing neurofeedback services.

Mentors: It is important to become familiar with the equipment used by your mentee in order to properly guide him/her in learning how to read trend screens, thermometers, reinforcement percentages and ratios, asymmetries, and the various components of neurofeedback sessions. This will help them assess progress with particular protocols.

Mentees: Your mentor should be able to look at neurofeedback sessions you have run on patients/clients and interpret what happened during a particular neurofeedback session as well as whether training objectives are being met.

Client/Patient Use of Medications

In the world of Real Estate, you will hear the phrase: Location, Location, Location. In the world of neurofeedback, you should keep in mind: Scope of Practice, Scope of Practice, Scope of Practice. How you approach discussions with clients/patients regarding medications is very important. If you do not prescribe medications to your patient or client, then your discussion regarding medications, medication use, and titrating off medications is best left to the prescriber.

It is fine to discuss the basics regarding medications and neurofeedback, but its use should be within your scope of practice or otherwise addressed in general terms. For example, patients/clients might come to you with the goal or getting off medications or using neurofeedback as an alternative to taking them.

It is generally safe and appropriate to discuss in general terms the following commonly asked questions by patient/clients regarding medication. Keep in mind that no two people are the same and they will not have the same side effects of medications, derive the same benefits from engaging in neurofeedback, nor have the same outcomes regarding medication reduction/titration.

Can neurofeedback help my disorder or symptoms if I don't use medications?
Using self-regulation training, many neurofeedback patients/clients have been able to alleviate various problematic symptoms and disorders.

Can neurofeedback help me reduce dosage or eliminate the use of medication?
Learning self-regulation through neurofeedback training may assist with reduction or elimination of medications when titration efforts are supervised closely by the prescriber.

How many sessions will it take before I can try to reduce or eliminate medication use?
Depending upon dosage, length of use, and individual physiology factors, the time necessary to reduce dosage or titrate off a particular medication will vary. Withdrawal effects must also be considered. This process should be guided by the prescriber.

What happens if I begin to reduce medication use and the symptoms return?
This is not uncommon. As noted above, the patient/client should be guided by the prescriber and the withdrawal symptoms should be discussed and monitored by the prescriber.

Explanations of Various Forms of Neurofeedback

There are various types of neurofeedback training modalities. Most commonly used are 1, 2, and 4-Channel traditional neurofeedback training, Z-Score training, sLORETA Neurofeedback, LENS, Infra Slow, etc.

Like other forms of biofeedback, neurofeedback training (NFT) uses monitoring devices to provide moment-to-moment information to an individual on the state of their physiological functioning. The characteristic that distinguishes NFT from other biofeedback is a focus on the central nervous system and the brain. NFT has its foundations in basic and applied neuroscience as well as data-based clinical practice. It takes into account behavioral, cognitive, and subjective aspects as well as brain activity.

NFT is preceded by an objective assessment of brain activity and psychological status. During training, sensors are placed on the scalp and then connected to sensitive electronics and computer software that detect, amplify, and record specific brain activity. Resulting information is fed back to the trainee virtually instantaneously with the conceptual understanding that changes in the feedback signal indicate whether or not the trainee's brain activity is within the designated range. Based on this feedback, various principles of learning, and practitioner guidance, changes in brain patterns occur and are associated with positive changes in physical, emotional, and cognitive states. Often the trainee is not consciously aware of the mechanisms by which such changes are accomplished although people routinely acquire a "felt sense" of these positive changes and often are able to access these states outside the feedback session.[V]

Infra-Slow and Infra-Slow Fluctuation Training are recent

V http://www.isnr.org/neurofeedback-introduction

developments in NF training and focused on the lowest frequencies in the brain below 0.1Hz. This type of training is performed on amplifiers designed to allow the lowest frequencies to pass through in order to provide feedback as they slowly increase and decrease over extended time periods involving minutes instead of milliseconds.[VI]

Low Energy Neurofeedback System (LENS) is a unique type of neurofeedback that nudges the brain out of maladaptive brainwave patterns it is stuck in by exposing the brain to a very high frequency signal at different locations, allowing it to restore homeostasis, to reset itself for optimal performance.[VI]

Z score neurofeedback measures EEG changes on the scalp in real time and compares then to a set of normative standard values. It then provides feedback to clients on how close or distant the actual EEG value is from the normative value. The EEG values used are derived from the neurometric dimensions used in most qEEG databases. Clients are typically training anywhere from 240 to over a thousand variables at once in five or more neurometric dimensions and receiving feedback from between two and nineteen locations across the scalp.

sLORETA neurofeedback goes one step further. During sLORETA neurofeedback, the EEG information from a client is collected from 19 locations on the scalp and special mathematical algorithm is used to localize current source anomalies in the cortex based on a normative reference. Consequently, the sLORETA algorithm estimates current source density in three-dimensional space intra-cortically. This allows for targeting specific regions of interest for feedback based on their deviation from normative activity. Users of sLORETA hope to gain more efficacy in training through enhanced specificity of training.

Expected Differences Between Eyes Closed/Eyes Open QEEG Brain Maps

If you are conducting QEEG Brain Maps, the most significant difference you should notice is the magnitude or power differences between eyes closed versus eyes opened maps.

VI http://www.brainneurofeedback.com/lens-neurofidback-faqs/

With eyes closed, the power distribution is Alpha (most prominent), followed by Theta, then Delta and Beta

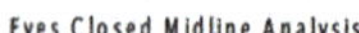

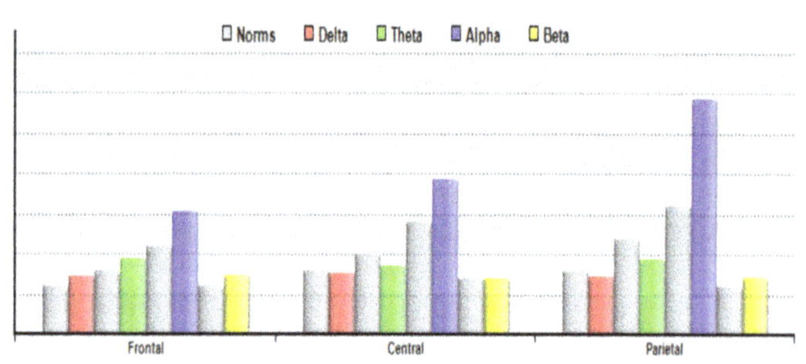

With Eyes opened, the power distribution is Delta, followed by Theta, then Alpha and Beta.

Eyes Open Midline Analysis

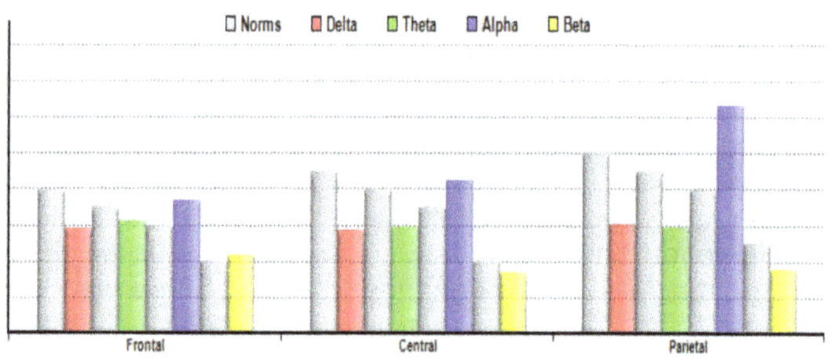

When do I use EC vs EO Training?

In most cases, neurofeedback providers would agree that training with eyes closed or eyes open is effective in enhancing self-regulation skills. Many will agree that eyes-closed training is beneficial when addressing anxiety, sleep problems, and pain; and eyes open is beneficial when addressing depression, attention, focus, and cognitive performance. Some practitioners only use eyes-open training; and many would agree that using eyes-open training is best when working with patients/clients who are under 16 years of age. Many young people have a difficult time trying to sit still with their eyes closed for 20-30 minutes. Some clients/patients do not tolerate eyes opened training while others do not tolerate eyes closed training. The bottom line is that there is no "Golden Rule" when it comes to using eyes closed vs. eyes opened neurofeedback. Practice and experience, in addition to client/patient differences, will guide you in your decisions.

Mentors: Your experience in working with various disorders and symptoms can help guide the mentee as when to use eyes closed versus eyes-open training.

Mentees: Eyes closed and eyes opened training are both effective. Some patients may not due well with eyes closed due to age or background trauma events. Always inquire of patients/ clients as to comfort level with eyes closed and work with your mentor to establish the most beneficial protocols.

Protocol Selection

Protocol selection in part may be determined by both the hardware and software that one uses, as well as protocols that have been used to focus on specific disorders and symptoms. Some equipment can only run one or two channel protocols, while others can run one, two, and four-channel protocols. Several pieces of neurofeedback equipment can run five or more channel training sessions, including full-cap training. Other pieces of equipment are preprogrammed to run one of several built-in protocols and there are limited choices.

Some pieces can run specialized neurofeedback protocols like Alpha Theta training while others cannot. It is for these reasons, among others, that it is important to talk with several manufacturers of neurofeedback equipment before purchasing one. Not all neurofeedback equipment can run the same types of neurofeedback (i.e., Z-Score, sLORETA), and therefore the types of protocols one may use can be limited.

When using QEEG Brain Maps, the map will guide you as to protocol set-up and in some cases, brain mapping systems provide the practitioner with recommend protocols based upon the map's findings. All of these options have value and benefits, but some have limitations as to what types of neurofeedback you can do. Appendix 14 provides a brief overview of basic neurofeedback training principles.

Commonly asked Questions by mentees include:

1. How do I know if/when to change protocols?
Changing protocols entails a variety of factors and theoretical frameworks that have emerged from pioneers in neurofeedback, today's leading practitioners, and what research supports. Some practitioners use the same protocol with a patient/client for 30-40 sessions and never make changes, while others use the same protocol 4-5 times and then deliberately switch to a new protocol. Some practitioners may train a patient/client with eyes closed for several sessions and then switch to eyes opened. Other practitioners switch protocols to address different problems/symptoms for which the patient/client is requesting help.

2. Explanation of protocols (why am I inhibiting and enhancing certain frequencies?)
Generally inhibiting or enhancing particular bandwidths is what produces the desired effects from neurofeedback training. This becomes easier to understand when one is using QEEG map- guided protocols because the map reveals what brain waves are too high or too low compared to normative data, and thus what brain waves might best be uptrained (enhanced) or down trained (inhibited).

In addition to uptraining or down-training amplitudes of various frequencies, many practitioners also train other neurometric dimensions such as coherence or phase using QEEG measures. In the absence of QEEG, there are some basic guidelines as to what bandwidths you take up or down and where (see Appendix 14 - Neurofeedback Training Guidelines).

In addition, there are scientific articles and case studies that are published and often include particular protocol settings and locations for which one might train to address particular disorders and/or symptoms (see https://www.isnr.org/resources and https://www.aapb.org/i4a/pages/index.cfm?pageid=3404).

Mentors: It is important to help guide mentees to understand protocols and how they work, protocol selection based upon disorders/symptoms, and how to build upon the knowledge they must have regarding traditional neurofeedback. Equipment, software, and skills level is critical in helping mentees select proper protocols. Scope of practice must be addressed regarding what the mentee is claiming/ offering/ attempting to address.

Mentees: Your mentor should be familiar with your equipment and the types of protocols you can incorporate into your neurofeedback training practice. With that knowledge, your mentor should be able to clearly explain what any protocol is doing, what brain wave functions a protocol is addressing, and why.

Home Training

Many practitioners engage in the rental of neurofeedback equipment to patients/clients, and clinical supervision of home training (the patient/client is taught how setup, prepare for, and run neurofeedback sessions at home on themselves or a family member).

Until you are BCIA Certified and feel confident about setting up neurofeedback protocols and brain wave training sessions without guidance or supervision, we encourage you to not engage in the use of home training with patients/clients. Home training presents many challenges. For example, the equipment and software you use should allow you to determine if the home trainee is running a session for the proper length of time, if electrodes are placed properly with good impedance, if an electrode comes loose, the length of the session, and other factors associated with the quality of the session.

There should be a contractual arrangement as to the frequency of sessions and costs including equipment lease, supplies being used, etc. The contractual arrangement should include what happens if the patient is non-compliant, if equipment breaks or malfunctions, technical support and the like.

What are the Costs of Being Mentored?

Many mentors charge a mentoring fee equivalent to what they would be charging a patient for a one hour therapy session or consult. Therefore, you will see a range of fees from as low as $50 and in some cases less, to $300 or more per hour. Take the time to explore and compare individual mentors to see which one is the best match for you. Keep in mind, familiarity with your equipment, use of brain maps, disorders /symptoms you are interested in working with, and types of neurofeedback you are interested in learning are important to take into consideration in your selection. If you cannot purchase equipment on your own and you don't have your own clinical practice with access to clients, you may be asking a different question. You are essentially asking to use equipment belonging to the mentor and to be able to practice on the mentor's patients/clients. This would be more of an internship. Carefully consider if you have a skill to trade in return for such an "internship". Could you perhaps work with patient/client records your mentor is assembling for research, could you do social media marketing to help offset the cost of the mentoring?

Mentoring Requirements

As noted previously, BCIA has specific mentoring requirements you must meet in order to complete your neurofeedback mentoring; however, in our experience, we find that mentoring sessions cover all types of material and issues from hardware and software, to treating specific disorders and proper record keeping.

Mentoring can begin when the mentee can demonstrate some basic competence with equipment and is only the time spent reviewing the actual work as outlined by BCIA. Primarily working on equipment issues or technical support is not mentoring and should not be included.

While BCIA's mentoring requirements are specific and clearly outlined, depending upon your skill, level of knowledge and experience in doing neurofeedback, your mentoring sessions may need to cover additional and practical skills in practicing neurofeedback. In many cases unusual clinical challenges may arise that require extensive review and discussions that go beyond basic mentoring requirements. This can involve some of the most valuable learning and transfer of information from a more experienced to a less experienced practitioner. A mentee's past clinical experience and the population they have worked with in the past may often define their methods and mindset from the outset but these perspectives and methods may need to be enhanced when working with neurofeedback and the population it may bring to their clinic. For instance, they may find that they encounter individuals with more physical or emotional trauma then they had dealt with in the past. Practicing neurofeedback may bring in more extreme cases than they are used to working with at the clinical level. This may confront them with their own deficits and experience in certain areas and require them to learn more and take more workshops on how to deal with these populations. Mentors should be able to directly assist them in learning more and be knowledgeable enough about the field to direct them to appropriate resources.

Documentation

Most practitioners already have a process by which they document progress notes or client/patient sessions. If you are a practicing clinician, then you will likely have a system in place. If not, your mentor may be able to make suggestions as to how to best document neurofeedback training sessions. In either case, you should document the particulars about your sessions; i.e., length of session, pre-post data, training sites and training parameters, client/patient response, unusual findings, etc. In addition, you should also be documenting the client's symptoms from session to session and carefully noting any changes. Often a standardized symptom tracking system of some type, either paper and pencil or computer based can be helpful. Since neurofeedback is EEG biofeedback, symptoms of interest are often physiological in nature and may differ from the domain of symptoms clinicians are accustomed to monitoring.

Drug Effects on EEG

Appendix 15 is a chart that addresses some of the basic drug groups effect on EEG. This is important to know and understand when you have clients/patients taking certain medications, especially those used to treat anxiety, depression, insomnia, ADD/ADHD and other mental health disorders. Recreational drugs such as Alcohol (including marijuana and CBD, which may be taken for medicinal purposes), also have effect on EEG; and may interfere with the quality and benefits of neurofeedback. These are important to know and understand when they are being used by the client/patient in conjunction with neurofeedback. EEG can be affected by medications and recreational drugs; and one should be familiar with the potential side effects a client/patient is experiencing as those side effects may worsen, as the brain begins to get healthy, during the course of neurofeedback.

An important part of mentoring involves training practitioners in how to talk to clients appropriately about the medications they use while staying within their scope of practice. Changes in medication can result in changes in symptoms that may incorrectly be attributed to neurofeedback training. They can also interfere with neurofeedback goals. Since this can lead to considerable confusion and distress for both client and practitioner alike, it is crucial to become familiar with drugs and their effects in a manner that practitioners are not accustomed to in their previous clinical role. In many cases the impact this has on new practitioners is unforeseen by them and overwhelming. Mentors should be thoroughly versed in this area and prepared to offer guidance.

Chapter Five – Helpful Hints and Information

Over the course of years of mentoring we have come across a variety of situations and experiences that are important to keep in mind. We have collected examples of some items to illustrate some of the points we will make.

Never Leave a Client/Patient Alone

Many of today's neurofeedback systems are set up to run a protocol without continuous monitoring. While this option provides opportunities and advantages for a practitioner to run multiple patients simultaneously, such freedom does not come without problems. Any number of things can happen during a session to cause it to go awry. For example, a patient falls asleep, an electrode comes loose, software locks up, a protocol adjustment needs to be made, etc. When events like this happen, there is usually a simple fix, but the practitioner needs to be present to assess the problem and correct it. It is not a problem to step out of the room temporarily to use the restroom, grab an important phone call, or get a drink of water; however, leaving a client/patient in a room unattended can be problematic and is never advised, especially for someone learning neurofeedback.

Next are examples of a neurofeedback session where the client/patient was left unattended by the practitioner. Within three minutes of the start of the first session, and six minutes of the second session, an electrode came loose, and the entire 30-minute session was run. In this example the client is training with a two-channel protocol but only one channel of data is present for feedback and review.

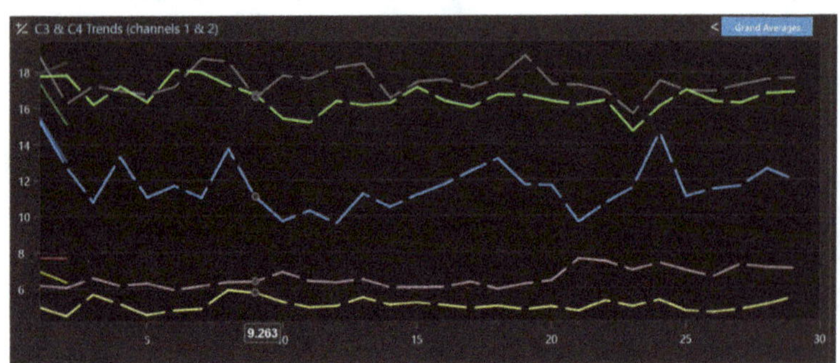
C3 & C4 Trends (channels 1 & 2)
Grand Averages
9.263

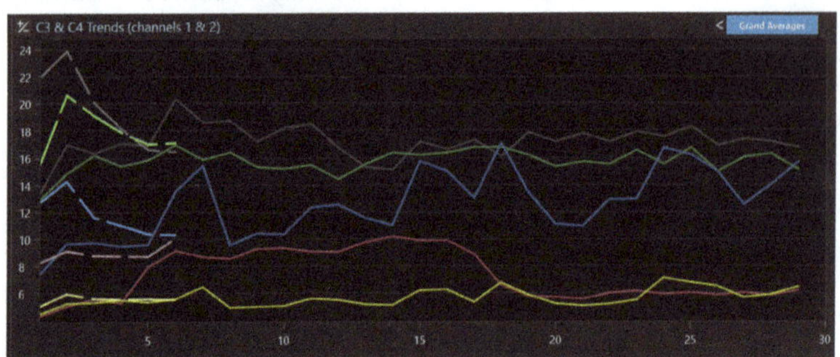
C3 & C4 Trends (channels 1 & 2)
Grand Averages

Electromagnetic Interference

Electromagnetic fields (EMF) are generated by a variety of electronics and electrical appliances. EMF is a physical field produced by electrically charged objects. It affects the behavior of charged objects in the vicinity of the field. The electromagnetic field extends indefinitely throughout space and describes the electromagnetic interaction.[VII]

We have spent hours with mentees helping them to troubleshoot problems when they run neurofeedback sessions and unusual EEG patterns show up on a neurofeedback session trend screen. Common examples of what can cause EMF and electrical interference with neurofeedback sessions when they are close to neurofeedback equipment include but are not limited to:

- Cell phones on the client/patient or within a few feet from him/her.
- Soda machines in an office.
- Telephone wiring boxes.
- Homes/office with old electrical wiring.
- Homes/offices with improper electrical grounding.
- Wi-Fi systems.
- Hand held talking devices

The session below on the right side of the screen demonstrates what can happen when a cell phone is left near or on the body of a client/patient.

VII http://en.wikipedia.org/wiki/electromagnetic_field

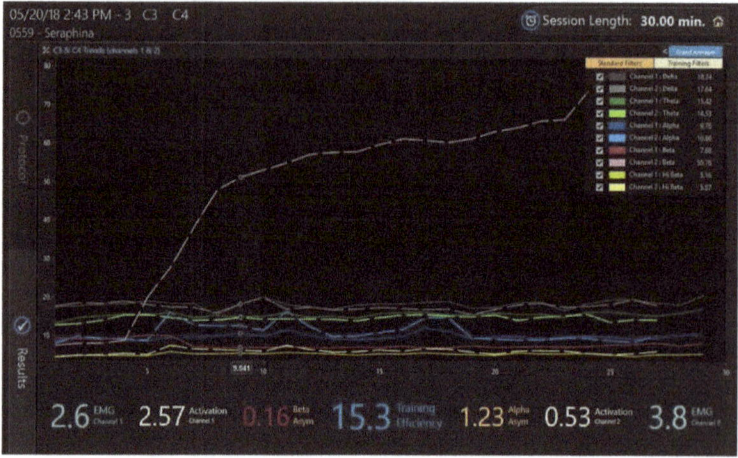

Learning to identify these problems and remediate them is unique to neurofeedback and each neurofeedback training system tends to be vulnerable to different forms of interference and artifact. This is another reason it can be valuable to work with a mentor that is familiar with your system. Knowing what problems can typically arise and how to quickly address them is crucial for maintaining efficiency and client confidence. Although many companies have excellent support, it is not always possible to get help when you require it the most. Each practitioner should be learning from their mentor which problems are likely to arise and how to address them.

Software Updates

Most neurofeedback devices are connected to and operated through software downloaded to a computer. To the best of our knowledge all neurofeedback systems are run in Microsoft Windows operating systems. At the time of this writing Windows 10 is the current system running Windows and related software. There are multiple documented examples across many neurofeedback software platforms in which a Windows update occurs and then neurofeedback software doesn't work. These updates can affect the drivers in your software and may require you to reboot your computer to get software running again. If a reboot doesn't fix the problem, you should call technical support for your brand of equipment.

Bad Connections

The human brain is an electrical system and the equipment we use to perform neurofeedback training is electrical as well. Good electrical connects (impedance) is essential in conducting neurofeedback sessions because we are continuously measuring the brain's electrical activity in order to provide it with accurate feedback. There are several situations that can negatively affect impedance. Some of the more common problems include:

Poor electrode placement (i.e., too little paste, excessive hair between the electrode and scalp).

Poor electrode connection (i.e., excessive hair product on the scalp such as hair spray, hair gel, hair dye). An example is a woman who was a neurofeedback trainee and participated in ballroom dancing contests. She dyed her hair black almost weekly which led to a buildup of dye on her scalp. Even after cleaning with NuPrep®, her impedance readings at best were always mediocre.

Bad Electrode (frayed or broken wires). Not all electrodes are made equal, but well-made electrodes can last up to a year or more when used, cleaned, and taken care of properly. Electrode wiring is fragile and it isn't difficult to break wires if they are not handled properly. Over time and with repeated use, wires and plugs will break. Therefore, it is recommended to always keep spare electrodes and ear clip on hand in case one breaks.

APPENDICES

Appendix 1 – Sample BCIA Mentoring Contract

BCIA EEG/Neurofeedback Mentoring Agreement

This letter constitutes the mentoring agreement between ______ (Mentee) and ______ (Mentor) for BCIA-EEG mentoring.

This process includes oversight and review of personal NFB training sessions, client/patient session review, clinical case reviews, and may also include learning, understanding and review of techniques, protocols, and equipment, chosen by the mentored candidate. This mentoring process will be based on BCIA recommendations and requirements as well as the BCIA Blueprint of Knowledge. Documentation of cases reviewed will be required in the form of case studies reviewed by ______. **As a candidate, you are expected to contact BCIA to inform them of your intent to become a candidate for mentoring, to register as a mentee, and acquire the necessary paperwork for mentoring.** Additionally, BCIA encourages mentees to work with other mentors. If you need to be mentored in a specific type of neurofeedback of which I do not use, please let me know and I will work with you to find the right mentor. BCIA Mentoring requires the following: 25 hours of mentoring (2 hours face-to-face), 10 Case Study presentations, 10 sessions of personal NFB demonstrating self-regulation, and 100 sessions of patient/client treatment (min 20 mins per session).

Mentees are expected to read, understand, and follow the BCIA Professional Standards and Ethical Principles of Biofeedback. Periodic performance reviews will be done between you and your Mentor using the BCIA Essential Skills List.

Schedule and Mentoring Times:

Mentoring will occur on a weekly, and/or as needed (PRN) basis. As Mentee, you may initiate phone calls and/or e-mails to set up mentoring times. Our standard time will be on ______ at ______.

Timeline for Mentoring:

Mentoring should be done in a consistent fashion and minimally include 25 hours (BCIA Mentoring requirement). This contract is good for up to 12 months and may be renewed if needed. The mentoring relations will begin ______ and will end ______. Experience indicates that those who make consistent efforts are most likely to complete the process. If the mentoring requirements are not completed, Mentor will sign off on the work completed. You may discuss options for a continuance of the mentoring relationship and this agreement, or you may seek another mentor to complete your requirements. If we agree that you will work with another mentor, BCIA must be notified of this change.

You are expected to carry liability insurance, and to use an Informed Consent for all persons you are training with neurofeedback.

Fees:

My charge for mentoring is ______ per hour. Payments may be made by mailing a check or via credit card. Sessions should be paid for at the time mentoring has occurred and may be paid in advance.

Type of Relationship:

BCIA mentoring is based upon a consultation model rather than a strict supervision model. This is not an agreement to provide clinical supervision to you, or to meet any licensing requirements. This agreement constitutes an "at will" arrangement and either party may end this agreement at any time. As your Mentor, ______ is not legally liable, or responsible for the patient care provided by you. Our relationship is that of "Consultant" or "Mentor". Please provide me with a copy of your intended informed consent information.

Conflict Resolution:

Within this mentoring relationship, it is possible for conflicts to arise. BCIA strongly supports and recommends conflict resolution through mediation if necessary.

Signing this agreement means both parties agree to pursue a respected mediator should a conflict arise that cannot be resolved between both parties. Both parties will divide the cost of mediation and will abide by the mediator's decision.

Record Keeping:

We will each document the contact hours for mentoring, the topics discussed, and review this log periodically to make sure we are in agreement of topics covered and issues addressed. Signatures below indicate acceptance and adherence to this agreement.

____
Candidate: Printed Name

____
Candidate: Signature

____
Date

____
Mentor Name & BCIA Certification#

____
Mentor Signature

____
Date

Appendix 2 - BCIA Professional Standards and Ethical Principles of Biofeedback

This document is designed to be a living document that will serve to guide your decisions and is meant to serve beside the ethical principles of your profession and within the laws of your state that govern health care. Please revisit this document time to time as it may change with updated information as needed.

Preamble

For the purposes of this document, the term BCIA professionals refers to BCIA certificants and those who have filed a formal application for BCIA certification.

Because the Biofeedback Certification International Alliance (BCIA) and its professionals are committed to the protection of human rights, they strive to maintain the dignity and worth of the individual while rendering service, conducting research, and teaching others. They operate within the BCIA Professional Standards and Ethical Principles (PSEP). They strive to provide the highest quality of service and carefully differentiate between empirically validated and experimental procedures. They hold themselves responsible for their actions and make every effort to protect their clients' welfare. Finally, they limit their services to those areas in which they have expertise and exemplify the values of competence, objectivity, freedom of inquiry, and honest communication.

The PSEP is intended to guide all BCIA professionals who commit themselves to adhere to these Principles as well as to the Principles stated in their licensing act. A copy of the PSEP will be provided to all BCIA certification applicants and will be available on the BCIA website. The PSEP are intended to educate and guide professionals to prevent ethical misconduct and should be applied with professional maturity.

The term biofeedback refers to all modalities for which we provide certification including, but not limited to, BVP, EEG or neurofeedback, electrodermal, EMG, HRV, respiration, and thermal biofeedback.

"Biofeedback is a process that enables an individual to learn how to change physiological activity for the purposes of improving health and performance. Precise instruments measure physiological activity such as brainwaves, heart function, breathing, muscle activity, and skin temperature.

These instruments rapidly and accurately 'feedback' information to the user. The presentation of this information — often in conjunction with changes in thinking, emotions, and behavior — supports desired physiological changes. Over time, these changes can endure without continued use of an instrument."

Purpose and Scope

The PSEP consist of guidelines for professional biofeedback practice that are not exhaustive and do not limit BCIA professionals' ethical responsibilities. They highlight areas in which ethical concerns often arise. For BCIA professionals who practice under a state and/or national licensing act, the PSEP are not meant to replace, but to confirm and reinforce, professional ethical guidelines.

1. The PSEP should be followed by BCIA certificants, applicants, and their staff who help provide biofeedback and related services.

2. BCIA professionals' ethical conduct is measured by the PSEP, state and/or national licensing acts, and the ethical guidelines of their professional membership organizations where applicable.

3. A violation of the PSEP may lead to disciplinary action or decertification. In some instances, such as sexual contact with a client, a criminal charge may result from breach of the PSEP and other professional guidelines for ethical practice.

A. Responsibility

In utilizing biofeedback, BCIA professionals adhere to the highest standards of their profession. They behave responsibly; accept responsibility for their behavior and its consequences; ensure that biofeedback is used appropriately; and strive to educate the public concerning the responsible use of biofeedback in treatment, training, and research. BCIA professionals are responsible for adhering to the ethical principles of their profession; the local, state and national laws relevant to their professional activities; and the PSEP.

1. As practitioners, BCIA professionals recognize their obligation to help clients acquire knowledge and skill through training that represents the best professional practice and that is delivered in the most cost-effective manner.

2. As teachers, BCIA professionals are committed to the advancement of knowledge. They encourage the free pursuit of learning by their students and present information objectively, accurately, and completely.

3. BCIA professionals guard against misuse of their influence since they realize that their professional services impact the lives of their clients and others.

4. BCIA professionals should only continue biofeedback services as long as their clients benefit from training. If their clients require an intervention that they are not qualified to provide, they should help them obtain these services and should never abandon them.

B. Competence

BCIA professionals recognize the boundaries of their competence and only use those biofeedback and adjunctive techniques in which they have expertise. They also recognize the proper limitations of biofeedback and inform all concerned parties about the clinical utility of particular procedures, possible negative effects, and whether the procedures are experimental or clinically verified. BCIA professionals maintain current knowledge of relevant basic and applied biofeedback research.

1. BCIA professionals should operate within applicable local, state, and national laws as well as in accordance with the ethical principles of their profession. BCIA certification is not a license to practice independently.

2. BCIA professionals who treat medical or psychological conditions must demonstrate professional competence as defined by applicable local, state, and national licensing/ credentialing laws. BCIA certification becomes invalid when a certificant's license is suspended, revoked, or not renewed due to an investigation of a complaint. Once suspended the individual will not be considered by BCIA for a re-certification based on providing services under supervision. A licensed professional who is suspended may only apply for recertification by BCIA after the license has been reinstated.

3. BCIA professionals who are not appropriately licensed or credentialed, and who wish to treat medical or psychological conditions, must acquire appropriate supervision according to applicable state and national laws and professional codes/regulations.

4. BCIA professionals must accurately describe their qualifications, training, experience, and/or specialty. They must only list degrees in an approved healthcare field earned from a regionally accredited academic institution when applying for BCIA certification. BCIA only certifies individuals who hold these degrees and only lists these credentials in its directory. When BCIA practitioners list BCIA certification in advertisements, business cards, directories, websites, and similar professional publications, that listing cannot include an unaccredited degree nor can it list a degree not related to health care.

C. Ethical Standards

BCIA professionals are sensitive to prevailing community norms and recognize that the violation of these standards may jeopardize the quality of their services, completion of professional responsibilities, and public trust in biofeedback.

1. BCIA professionals will only charge for services actually provided by them or by those under their legal supervision. In billing third party

payers, practitioners will comply with the rules and regulations of the third-party payer, including clearly specifying which services the practitioner provided directly and which were supervised, and providing information regarding their qualifications (e.g., degree, license, and certification).

2. BCIA professionals will clarify any potential or actual conflict of interest that exists when serving clients, conducting training or research, or when engaged in any other professional activity (such as a workshop in which presenters recommend their own product).

3. BCIA professionals will obtain written informed consent from clients for all assessment and treatment procedures, billings and fee collections, and procedures to protect confidentiality, as well as conditions that limit confidentiality.

4. BCIA professionals will obtain written informed consent from clients for all experimental treatment applications. To distinguish experimental and clinically validated procedures is difficult and requires familiarity with related documents.

D. Multiculturalism and Diversity

1. BCIA professionals are encouraged to recognize that, as cultural beings, they may hold attitudes and beliefs that can detrimentally influence their perceptions of and interactions with individuals who are different from themselves ethnically, racially, in sexual orientation, or gender identity.

2. BCIA professionals are encouraged to recognize the importance of multicultural sensitivity/responsiveness to, knowledge of, and understanding about individuals who are different ethnically, racially, in sexual orientation, or gender identity.

3. As educators, BCIA professionals are encouraged to employ the constructs of multiculturalism and diversity in education.

4. Culturally sensitive researchers are encouraged to recognize the importance of conducting culture-centered and ethical research among persons from diverse ethnic, linguistic, racial, sexual orientation, or gender identity backgrounds.

5. BCIA professionals are encouraged to apply culturally appropriate skills in clinical and other biofeedback practices.

6. BCIA professionals are encouraged to use positive motivational change processes to support culturally informed organizational (policy) development and practices.

7. BCIA professionals regularly engage in professional reading and education (both online and face to face) on multiculturalism and diversity, keeping up to date on current standards and research.

E. Public Statements

BCIA professionals recognize that all public statements, announcements of services and products, advertising, and promotional activities concerned with biofeedback should help the public make informed choices. Statements about biofeedback must be based on scientifically verifiable information, including recognition of the limits and uncertainties of such data. BCIA professionals must accurately represent their qualifications, affiliations, and positions, and must not mislead the public.

1. BCIA professionals shall accurately represent the efficacy of biofeedback procedures for all disorders or conditions being treated.

2. BCIA professionals must use accurate information in statements about biofeedback when providing services, marketing a product, and in all other professional activities. They consider the context and source requesting information when making a public statement and guard against misrepresentation.

3. BCIA professionals recognize that they may have personal interests when they promote biofeedback activities and agree that these interests must be superseded by professional objectivity, concern for

clients' welfare, and the PSEP and the standards of other professional societies to which they belong. When a question arises as to their objectivity, they seek professional guidance from appropriate professional sources like BCIA and their professional associations.

4. Announcements and listing of services and training offered by BCIA professionals, such as service directory listings, letterheads, business cards, and marketing brochures and websites, should be accurate and designed in a professional manner, and should adhere to the guidelines of their professional associations.

F. Confidentiality

BCIA professionals protect the confidentiality of their clients' data. They may only release information with the written consent of the client or the client's legal representative, or when nondisclosure would endanger the client or others.

1. BCIA professionals specify in advance the legal limits of confidentiality to clients, particularly when collecting fees and complying with mandated reporting laws that concern abuse or neglect. Confidentiality applies to clients in treatment, students in training, and research participants.

2. Client records are stored and destroyed in ways that maintain confidentiality. BCIA professionals will keep records for the time required by applicable national and state laws.

G. Protection of Client Rights and Welfare

BCIA professionals protect the welfare of clients, students, research participants, and other groups with whom they work. They inform all consumers of their rights, provide them with a written statement of these rights, fully inform them as to the purpose and nature of procedures to be implemented, and assure that clients' rights are not abridged.

1. Sexual intimacy with current clients, trainees, supervisees, and research subjects is prohibited. BCIA professionals should follow the

applicable guidelines of state/national law and their professional associations regarding when sexual intimacy is permissible after termination of a professional relationship.

2. Professionals adhere to the highest standards of infection mitigation to protect clients and staff. Practitioners are responsible to learn and follow reasonable disinfection standards applicable to biofeedback instruments, sensors, and office environments.

3. In attaching biofeedback sensors, professionals assure that the privacy and rights of the client are protected and respect the feelings and sensitivities of their clients. Caution and common sense are required whenever an applicant or certificant has physical contact with clients. Any physical contact requires the permission of the client. Touching of sensitive body parts, such as breasts or genitals, is not acceptable in biofeedback practice, with the exception of a medical exam or medical treatment provided by a licensed medical practitioner.

4. Special care is taken to protect the rights of children when providing biofeedback training or conducting research. Wherever possible, BCIA professionals should seek children's agreement to participate in these activities.

5. BCIA professionals do not discriminate against or refuse services to anyone on the basis of sex, sexual orientation, gender identity, race, religion, disability, or national origin.

H. Professional Relationships

BCIA professionals recognize the interdisciplinary nature of biofeedback and respect the competencies of colleagues in all professions. They strive to act in accordance with the obligations of the organizations with which they and their colleagues are associated. They:

1. Should only treat medical disorders if clients have first received a medical evaluation and/or are under the care of a physician.

2. Should strive to be objective in their professional judgment of colleagues and to maintain good professional relationships even when opinions differ.

3. Should avoid multiple relationships with their clients that could impair their professional judgment or increase the risk of exploitation, and must never exploit clients, students, supervisees, employees, research participants, or third party payers.

I. Research with Humans and Animals

BCIA professionals conduct research to advance understanding of human behavior, to improve human health and welfare, and to advance science. They carefully consider alternative research methods and assure that in the conduct of research the welfare of research participants (human and animal) is protected.

All researchers will adhere to state and national regulations and the professional standards of their profession with regard to the conduct of research. Research involving humans may be subject to regulation by local institutional review boards and to state and/or national regulations.

Animal research may be subject to local institutional animal care and use committees and must comply with state and national policies on the use of animals.

1. The results of research will be released in a manner which accurately reflects research results and only when the findings have satisfied widely-accepted scientific criteria. Any limitations regarding factors such as sampling bias, small samples, and limited follow-up, will be explicitly stated. All descriptive materials distributed regarding clinical practice will be factual and straightforward.

2. The individual researcher is responsible for the establishment and maintenance of acceptable ethical practice in research. The investigator is also responsible for the ethical treatment of research participants by collaborators, assistants, students, and employees, all of whom also incur similar obligations. Information obtained about

research participants during the course of an investigation should be confidential. When the possibility exists, that others may obtain access to such information, ethical research practice requires that this possibility, together with the plans to protect confidentiality, be explained to the participants as part of the procedure for obtaining informed consent.

3. Ethical practice requires that the investigator inform participants of all features of the research that might be reasonably expected to influence their willingness to participate and to explain all other aspects of the research about which the participant inquires. BCIA professionals protect participants from physical and psychological discomfort, harm, and danger. If the risk of such consequences exist, investigators are required to inform the participant of that fact, secure informed consent before proceeding, and take all possible measures to minimize distress. A research procedure may not be used if it is likely to cause serious and lasting harm to participants.

As participants' risk increases, so does the responsibility of the researcher to protect the research participants. Written informed consent or a verbal and written summary of the research is customary for most kinds of non-survey research (including a signature by the research participant in both cases).

4. The investigator must respect an individual's freedom to decline to participate in research or to discontinue participation at any time. The obligation to protect this freedom requires special vigilance when the investigator has power over the participant. When a prospective participant is a minor, investigators should seek the child's assent.

5. After research data are collected, the investigator must fully debrief participants about the nature of the study. When scientific or human values justify delaying or withholding information, the investigator acquires a special responsibility to assure that the participant is not harmed.

Adherence to Professional Standards

BCIA professionals should be knowledgeable about efficacious interventions and adhere to the professional standards associated with these techniques.

Additional Standards

BCIA professionals who hold a state or national license/credential should adhere to the guidelines of the relevant professional licensing act. Additional guidance can be found in the ethical standards of organizations like the American Psychological Association, American Psychiatric Association, the American Nurses Association, the American Physical Therapy Association, the American Medical Association, the American Dental Association, the American College of Sports and Rehabilitation, the American Academy of Physical Medicine and Rehabilitation, and their international counterparts.

Ethics Complaint Procedures

When BCIA receives a written complaint about the ethical conduct of a BCIA certificant or applicant, BCIA's Executive Director will record the complaint and will write a letter to the complainant that will describe BCIA's role in ethics cases, direct the complainant to directly discuss the complaint with the provider (certificant or applicant), and if requested by the complainant, identify state and/or national regulatory agencies with jurisdiction. Since BCIA's approach to ethical issues is educational, BCIA will not recommend that complainants contact these agencies nor will it represent complainants before these agencies.

BCIA will not intervene in complaints about manufacturer or vendor products, services, or sales practices as these issues do not concern certification and corporations are not BCIA professionals.

While BCIA encourages certificants to first discuss ethical concerns with their colleagues, certificants may directly contact appropriate regulatory agencies. If an agency declares that a complaint lacks merit, is frivolous, or is malicious, BCIA will defer to the agency to discipline the complainant.

The BCIA Board of Directors will periodically review and update the PSEP. Thereafter, BCIA professionals shall be required to adhere to the revised PSEP. Comment is invited. Individuals desiring more information about these Principles may contact BCIA.

Related Documents and Acknowledgments

1. Biofeedback Alliance and Nomenclature Task Force (2008).
2. Regulations for the protection of human research subjects (45 CFR46 and 56 FR 28003) (Federal Regulations).
3. Humane care and use of animals (A 343401) (Federal Regulations).
4. Hagedorn, D. (2014). Infection risk mitigation for biofeedback providers. Biofeedback, 42(3), 93-95.
5. G. Tan, F. Shaffer, R. Lyle, & I. Teo (Eds.). Evidence based practice in biofeedback and neurofeedback (3rd ed.). Wheat Ridge, CO: Association for Applied Psychophysiology and Biofeedback.

We thank the Association for Applied Psychophysiology and Biofeedback, whose Ethical Principles were modified and adapted for these Principles. Original version adopted by BCIA Board of Directors, August 26, 1990.

1st revision prepared by John G. Carlson, Adopted by the BCIA Board of Directors, October 14, 1999.
2nd revision prepared and adopted by the BCIA Board of Directors, March 24, 2002.
3rd revision prepared and adopted by the BCIA Board of Directors, April 5, 2004.
4th revision prepared and adopted by the BCIA Board of Directors, April 1, 2005.
5th revision prepared and adopted by the BCIA Board of Directors, August 26, 2009.
6th revision prepared and adopted by the BCIA Board of Directors, May 18, 2015.
7th revision prepared and adopted by the BCIA Board of Directors, October 6, 2015.
8th revision prepared and adopted by the BCIA Board of Directors, January 29, 2016.
9th revision prepared and adopted by the BCIA Board of Directors, May 2, 2016.

Appendix 3 - Essential Skills List for Neurofeedback

NEUROFEEDBACK ESSENTIAL SKILLS LIST

A beginning neurofeedback practitioner should be able to demonstrate mastery of the following basic skills, as attested by their BCIA-approved Mentor who will initial each item as completed.

Client/Patient Orientation

___1. In layman's language, explain to a new client EEG biofeedback, self-regulation concepts, and operant conditioning of brainwave activity.
___2. Explain the major stages in the neurofeedback treatment/training process, from initial intake and assessment to progress monitoring and reporting.
___3. Explain client's role and responsibilities in the neurofeedback process.
___4. At initial session, explain how the neurofeedback session process and equipment works, including:

- Purpose and steps involved in skin preparation.
- Steps in electrode attachment and selection of site placements; assure client about safety of "sensors"/ electrodes.
- Meaning of primary features of the feedback screens and concepts of amplitude and frequency and/or z-scores.
- Relationship between client activity and on-screen feedback changes.
- Session recording and progress monitoring screens.

___5. Obtain written client permission for treatment/training using a thorough Informed Consent form.

Intake, Assessment and Protocol Selection

___1. Document a thorough client symptom and medication history and gather background information relevant to treatment/training goals.

___2. Provide a thorough EEG baseline assessment, using the following skills:

- Perform correct measurements to name and locate on the scalp each of the International 10-20 System electrode placement sites .
- Properly prepare scalp and ears and attach electrodes to selected assessment sites or attach an electrode cap if doing a full-cap quantitative EEG.
- Correctly perform all steps to collect a qEEG recording or multi-channel EEG assessment: checking impedances, removing artifact, and collecting eyes-open and eyes-closed data .
- Demonstrate basic understanding of a qEEG assessment report, as well as the most commonly reported components of qEEG databases (absolute power, relative power, phase, coherence, z-score comparisons, etc.).
- Identify recordings indicating spike and wave activity requiring consultation with a neurologist or qEEG expert.
- Use all intake, psychometric, and baseline EEG assessment data to select target electrode placement sites and montages for neurofeedback treatment/training.
- Select an initial neurofeedback protocol and explain rationale to client.

Use and Maintenance of Neurofeedback Equipment

___1. Demonstrate thorough knowledge of operation of neurofeedback equipment of choice:

- Make correct hardware connections and start hardware.
- Make correct electrode connections to the hardware.
- Identify and remove (or control for) sources of common artifacts in the raw EEG signal.
- Troubleshoot common equipment failures according to manufacturer's recommendations.

___2. Demonstrate thorough knowledge of appropriate software for selected equipment:

- Accurately select, install, and run neurofeedback treatment/ training software.
- Identify components, applications, and limitations of selected software package.

Neurofeedback Session Management and Reporting

___ 1. Conduct neurofeedback treatment/training sessions involving the following procedures:

- Provide initial orientation and instructions to client at first treatment/training session.
- Prior to subsequent sessions, query client (and/or parent) verbally and/or via pre-session questionnaire on client's positive and negative reactions to previous session.
- Maintain basic hygiene procedures in attaching (and cleaning) electrodes.
- Remind client of the training objectives for session and their role in attending to and responding to feedback.
- Start treatment/training software program, set up selected protocol parameters, and run basic feedback functions.
- As appropriate, set initial training thresholds and adjust as needed.
- Identify and remove sources of artifact appearing in session recordings.
- Monitor session recordings and provide coaching and supplemental verbal feedback to client during sessions, as appropriate.
- Save session data per equipment guidelines and review session results with client.
- Assign homework to client that supports and supplements session training goals.
- Consult with client's prescribing physician and/or providers of other concurrent treatments as necessary to avoid treatment complications and maximize treatment outcomes.
- Identify as soon as possible in the treatment/training process when neurofeedback is not working for a client; identify cause(s) for lack of progress; make necessary protocol or other training program adjustments; or, when necessary, recommend termination of neurofeedback.
- In collaboration with client, determine when neurofeedback treatment/training goals have been met and mutually plan for treatment termination and follow-up.
- Conduct all aspects of neurofeedback treatment and training in accordance with BCIA, AAPB and ISNR codes of ethical practice.

___ 2. Maintain orderly and up-to-date client files, including
- Session-by-session training records, significant session events and client comments.
- Changes in client medication, significant life changes, allergies, etc. that may impact treatment/training results.
- Reports of consultations with other treatment providers, family members, teachers, etc.

Use of Supplemental Therapeutic and Training Modalities

1. ___Demonstrate ability to establish positive, constructive relationships with clients and their family members, using basic counseling and/or communication skills.
2. ___Document adequate training and demonstrate skills required to use appropriate counseling/therapy methods to supplement neurofeedback with clients having mental health diagnoses, if applicable.
3. ___Document adequate training in use of neurofeedback protocols. Demonstrate ability to select appropriate clients for specific neurofeedback protocols, as well as apply appropriate therapy methods when using these protocols.
4. ___Document adequate understanding of other neuromodulation modalities (such as HRV biofeedback, AVS, CES, etc.) for use in conjunction with neurofeedback, and demonstrate ability to select and use appropriate adjunctive modalities with individual clients, if applicable.

I attest that this work has been completed for:

______________________ ________________________________

Name of Candidate for BCIA Certification

Signature of the Mentor: ________________________ Date: _______

Printed Name of Mentor____________________ BCIA #:___________

If using more than 1 mentor, please make copies of this document for each mentor to complete.

Note: More than one mentor may be used. Please submit this form for each mentor.

Appendix 4 – BCIA Mentoring Documentation Log

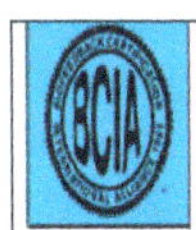

BCIA Mentoring for Neurofeedback Certification
Time/Activities Log Form

Applicant ____________________________________

Mentor_________________________ **Certification#** _____________

The log below lists the specific dates, times and descriptions of mentoring activities being presented for certification.

Date	25 Contact Hours	Description of Mentoring Activities	10 Personal Sessions	100 Patient/ Client Sessions	10 Case Confer-ences

Contact Hours Completed with Mentor: ________ **Hours**

I attest that the mentoring hours listed above are accurate.

BCIA Mentor Signature ______________________ **Date:** ________

Applicant Signature _________________________ **Date:** ________

Appendix 5 - BCIA Core Reading List

The following list of reading sources is suggested for individuals who are preparing for Board Certification in Neurofeedback. Each of these books provides basic coverage of most rubric areas covered by the BCIA Blueprint of Knowledge Statements for Board Certification in Neurofeedback. The remaining sources below provide additional information that may not be fully covered in one of the basic texts.

1. Biofeedback Certification International Alliance (2015) Blueprint of Knowledge Statements for Board Certification in Neurofeedback.
2. Biofeedback Certification International Alliance (2016). Professional Standards and Ethical Principles of Biofeedback.
3. Collura, T.F. (2014). Technical foundations of neurofeedback. New York: Routledge.
4. Demos, J. N. (2005). Getting started with neurofeedback. New York: W. W. Norton & Company.
5. ISNR Practice Guidelines for Neurofeedback (2013).
6. LaVaque, T. J., Hammond, D. C., Trudeau, D., Monastra, V., Perry, J., Lehrer, P., Matheson, D., & Sherman, R. (2002, December). Template for developing guidelines for the evaluation of the clinical efficacy of psychophysiological evaluations. Applied Psychophysiology and Biofeedback, 27(4), 273-281.
7. Pigott, H. E., DeBiase, L., Bodenhamer-Davis, E, & Davis, R. E. (2013) The evidence-base for neurofeedback as a reimbursable healthcare service to treat attention deficit/hyperactivity disorder.
8. Soutar, R. & Longo, R. (2011). Doing neurofeedback: An introduction. San Rafael, CA: ISNR Research Foundation.
9. Tan, G., Shaffer, F., Lyle, R., and Teo, I. (2016). Evidence-based practice in biofeedback and neurofeedback - 3rd edition. Wheat Ridge, CO: AAPB.
10. Thompson, M. & Thompson, L. (2003) or the 2nd edition (2015). The neurofeedback book. Wheat Ridge, CO: Association for Applied Psychophysiology and Biofeedback.

Appendix 6 - Recommended Reading List and Supplemental Reading List

The following sources are provided for those seeking additional information beyond the introductory knowledge level required for the Neurofeedback Certification Exam.

Technical Aspects of Neuromodulation

1. Cannon, R.L. (2012). Low resolution brain electromagnetic tomography (LORETA). Basic concepts and clinical applications. Corpus Christi, TX: BMed Press.
2. Coben, R. & Evans, J.R. (Eds.) (2011). Neurofeedback and neuromodulation techniques and applications. London: Academic Press.
3. Hammond, D.C. & Gunkelman, J. (2011). The art of artifacting, Vol. 2. Corpus Christi, TX: BMed Press.
4. Kropotov, J.D. (2009). Quantitative EEG, event-related potentials and neurotherapy. London: Academic Press.
5. Thatcher, R.W. (2012). Handbook of Quantitative Electroencephalography, ANIpublishing, Inc., St. Petersburg, Fl 33772.

Recommended and Supplemental Reading List

1. Amen, D. G. (2005). Making a good brain great. New York: Three Rivers Press.
2. Amen, D. G. (1998). Change your brain, change your life: The breakthrough program for conquering anxiety, depression, obsessiveness, anger and impulsiveness. New York: Three Rivers Press.
3. Begley, S. (2007). Train your mind, change your brain: How a new science reveals our extraordinary potential to transform ourselves. New York: Ballentine Books.
4. Carter, R. (2009). The human brain book. NY: DK Publishing.
5. Doidge, N. (2007). The Brain That Changes Itself: Stories of Personal Triumph from the Frontiers of Brain Science. NY: Penguin Press.
6. Doidge, N. (2016). The brain's way of Healing: Remarkable Discoveries and Recoveries from the Frontiers of Neuroplasticity. NY: Penguin Press.

7. Goldberg, E. (2009). The executive brain: Frontal lobes and the civilized mind. Revised and Expanded. USA: Oxford University Press.
8. Kotulak, R. (1996). Inside the brain: Revolutionary discoveries of how the mind works. Kansas City, MO: Andrews McMeel Publishing.
9. Ledoux, J. (1996). The emotional brain: the mysterious underpinnings of emotional life NY: Touchstone.
10. Moyers, B. (1993). Healing and the mind. New York: Doubleday.
11. Robbins, Jim. (2000). A symphony in the brain. New York: Grove Hills.
12. Soutar, R. (2017). The automatic self: transformation & transcendence through brainwave training. Lincoln, NE: iUniverse.

Appendix 7 - Informed Consent

Below is a sample of an Informed Consent form.

The purpose of this form is to obtain your voluntary consent to participate in one or more methods of quantitative electroencephalography (QEEG) brain mapping, peripheral biofeedback, neurofeedback, other forms of relaxation and stress reduction interventions, and to disclose potential benefits and risks associated with these interventions. (Business Name) provides various educational interventions, assessment protocols, and health care services, a few of which are still considered by some to be experimental.

QEEG Brain Mapping

To determine an appropriate neurofeedback training plan, a QEEG performed by (Business Name) using the (Company) expert referential database system will be conducted.

(Business Name) will assess your need for having a QEEG. To engage in neurofeedback, you will be required to have a QEEG assessment. In other instances, to help verify a disorder, your doctor, or another health care professional, may recommend you have a QEEG. A QEEG consists of placing a cap on your head with 20 electrodes/sensors. Each site will be cleansed, and a special gel will be placed under each sensor to insure proper conductivity to read your brainwaves. Preparation and the assessment procedure take approximately 1 hour.

Benefits: QEEG may help me further understand and/or confirm the problems/symptoms, disorders, and/or diagnosis for which I am seeking assessment and health care services.

Side Effects/Risks: QEEG may result in my feeling anxious/ apprehensive, and/or uncomfortable during the procedure, and sad/ disappointed regarding findings from the procedure. The cap may cause you to have a mild headache.

Forensic Services: QEEG brain mapping for purposes of neurofeedback is not a medical procedure and is not done at (Business Name) for purposes of medical diagnosis. Data collected is not done in a manner that meets the **Daubert** criteria for admissibility of evidence in court. (Business Name) does not provide forensic services or diagnosis for TBI. We do not accept invitations for depositions. Those seeking a diagnosis for TBI or any other diagnosable medical or mental disorder should seek services of an appropriate health care professional such as a physician or a forensic neuropsychologist. Your signature below indicates you agree not to request or seek such services from us presently or in the future, or through third parties such as legal counsel or insurance companies.

Client/Patient Rights. You have the right to:

- Decide not to receive QEEG brain mapping services from us. If you wish, we can provide you with the names of other qualified QEEG providers.
- End the QEEG at any time.
- Ask questions about protocol and procedures used during the QEEG procedure, and to ask questions about QEEG techniques if you feel unsure of them.
- Have all that you say treated confidentially and be informed of state law placing limitations on confidentiality in the QEEG relationship. Under certain circumstances, we are required by law to reveal information obtained during a QEEG assessment to other persons or agencies without your permission. Also, we are not required to inform you of our actions in this regard. These situations are as follows: (a) if you threaten bodily harm or death to yourself or another person, we are required by law to notify the victim and appropriate law enforcement agencies; (b) if a court of law issues a subpoena; (c) if you are having a QEEG or being tested by a court of law, the results of the QEEG assessment must be revealed to the court; (d) if you have given us information concerning non-accidental injury and neglect to minors or incompetent adults; or (e) if you are in the process of filing a workman's compensation claim or file such in the future.

Equipment/Software: QEEG measures will involve the use of the. (Business Name) software and hardware (equipment type). (Business Name) products are FDA registered. QEEG maps are produced using (report system).

Neurofeedback Training

Neurofeedback involves several electrodes/sensors being placed on the scalp and earlobes. The sensors detect brain wave activity including alpha, beta, delta, and theta brainwaves. Individual brain waves are measured and displayed on a computer screen revealing your brainwave activity. Through instruction you can learn to train down or train up certain brain waves associated with stress management, attention, cognitive and/or emotional deficits, and related disorders. In some cases, neurofeedback must be considered as experimental. Treatments last from 10–30 minutes and may occur two or more times per week for an average of 30–40 sessions, and in some cases, more than 40 sessions.

Benefits: Neurofeedback (NFB) is known to assist individuals by decreasing symptoms associated with brain and central nervous system dysfunction. Other benefits include the possibility of reducing problem behaviors and increasing peak performance. In many cases, neurofeedback is experimental when used to a treat certain disorders. Please feel free to ask for a more detailed explanation regarding your problem area or treatment interest.

Side Effects/Risks: Neurofeedback will not interfere with most other treatments. Neurofeedback has few side effects when administered properly. The most common side effects of neurofeedback include improved sleep, more awareness of dreams, feeling calmer, more energetic, and more focused. Temporary side effects such as headaches, insomnia, anxiety, feeling giddy, agitated, or irritated may occur during or right after a neurofeedback session. However, these side effects can be adjusted and eliminated immediately in most cases. It is also possible that you might fall asleep during or after neurofeedback sessions.

Client Rights. You have the right to:

- Decide not to receive neurofeedback services from us. If you wish, we can provide you with the names of other Board Certified neurofeedback providers in your area.
- End neurofeedback sessions at any time.
- Ask questions about protocols and procedures used during neurofeedback training, and to ask questions about techniques if you feel unsure of them.
- Have all that you say treated confidentially and be informed of state law placing limitations on confidentiality in the neurofeedback relationship. Under certain circumstances, we are required by law to reveal information obtained during training to other persons or agencies without your permission. Also, we are not required to inform you of our actions in this regard. These situations are as follows: (a) if you threaten bodily harm or death to yourself or another person, we are required by law to notify the indicated victim and appropriate law enforcement agencies; (b) if a court of law issues a subpoena; (c) if you are being treated with neurofeedback, at the direction of an attorney or medical doctor for legal purposes, the results of the training or tests must be revealed to the court; (d) if you have given us information concerning non-accidental injury and neglect to minors or incompetent adults; or (e) if you are in the process of filing a workman's compensation claim or have plans to file such in the future.

Equipment/Software: Neurofeedback treatment will involve the use of the (Business Name) software and hardware (equipment type). (Business Name) products are FDA registered.

Other Methods: Other treatment methods may not work as rapidly as the methods and modalities described above. Alternative methods of treatment and/or therapy include traditional medical treatments, medications, the use of supplements, the use of relaxation techniques, and/or group and individual therapy.

Choosing the Right Intervention: The interventions described above are voluntary, not mandatory. You will not be pressured to participate. You may withdraw from or stop receiving neurofeedback training sessions at any time without consequence.

Consent

I voluntarily consent to participate in and undergo the assessment and/or intervention methods and modalities described above. I understand that I am free to withdraw my consent and to discontinue participation in the interventions/modalities/methods described above at any time. The natural consequences and potential risks and benefits have been fully explained to me by (Business Name).

Permission

My signature below indicates that I have read, reviewed and understand this informed consent (and/or I have had the form and its contents read to me and explained to me), and I consent to participate in the procedures described above. I understand I may ask questions at any time, and may request to stop interventions at any time.

I have read and understand my rights.

____

Client Signature

____

Date

Appendix 8 - Client Bill of Rights and Responsibilities Regarding Biofeedback and Neurofeedback

Below is a sample of a Client/Patient Bill of Rights and Responsibilities form.

We want to encourage you, as a client of (Business Name), to speak openly with your clinical provider, take part in your assessment and treatment choices, and promote your own safety and well-being by being well informed and involved in your biofeedback (BFB) and neurofeedback (NFB) treatment services. You are encouraged to think of yourself as a partner in your care, and therefore to know your rights as well as your responsibilities during your course of treatment. (Business Name) provides various educational interventions, assessment protocols, and treatment services, a few of which are still considered, by some, to be experimental.

Client Rights:

- You have the right to receive considerate, respectful, and compassionate treatment in a safe setting, free from all forms of abuse, neglect, or mistreatment, regardless of your age, gender, race, national origin, religion, sexual orientation, gender identity, or disabilities. You have the right to inquire about and discuss ethical issues related to your care at all times, and to voice your concerns about the care you receive.
- You have the right to be told by your treatment provider about your diagnosis and possible prognosis, the benefits and risks of treatment, and the expected outcome of treatment. You have the right to give written informed consent before any non-emergency procedure begins, and to understand the costs of assessment and treatment before you begin.
- You, your family, and friends with your permission, have the right to participate in decisions about your treatment, including the right to refuse/withdraw from treatment.
- You have the right to decide not to receive BFB/NFB treatment from us. If you wish, we can provide you with the names of other BFB/NFB providers in your area.

- You have the right to ask questions about protocol and procedures used during all BFB/NFB sessions, and to ask questions about NFB/BFB techniques. You have the right to prevent the use of certain training techniques if you feel unsure of them, and to participate in setting goals and evaluating progress towards meeting them.
- You have the right to have all that you say treated confidentially and be informed of state law placing limitations on confidentiality in the NFB/BFB relationship. Under certain circumstances, we are required by law to reveal information obtained during NFB/BFB to other persons or agencies without your permission. Also, we are not required to inform you of our actions in this regard. These situations are as follows: (a) if you threaten bodily harm or death to yourself or another person, we are required by law to notify the intended victim and appropriate law enforcement agencies; (b) if a court of law issues a subpoena; (c) if you are in NFB/BFB training or being tested by a court of law, the results of the treatment or tests must be revealed to the court; (d) if you have given us information concerning non-accidental injury and neglect to minors or incompetent adults; or (e) if you are in the process of filing a workman's compensation claim or file such in the future.

Client Responsibilities—You Are Expected to:

1. Provide complete and accurate information, including your full name, address, home telephone number, date of birth, and employer when it is required.
2. Provide complete and accurate information about your health and medical history, including present condition, past illnesses, hospital stays, medicines, vitamins, herbal products, and any other matters that pertain to your health, including perceived safety risks.
3. Ask questions when you do not understand information or instructions. If you believe you cannot follow through with your treatment plan, you are responsible for telling your treatment provider. You are responsible for outcomes if you do not follow the treatment plan.

1. Provide complete and accurate information about your finances and your ability to pay your fees in accordance with the arrangement you established previously with (Business Name).
2. Set and keep appointments with your provider and be on time for your appointments. **Appointments cancelled without at least 24-hour notice are subject to a $50 charge**.
3. Help plan your therapy goals and keep your NFB/BFB provider informed of your progress toward meeting your goals.
4. Inform your NFB/BFB provider of any problems you have which may influence your progress or which may be potentially harmful to yourself or others.
5. Notify (Business Name) if you intend to discontinue training.

I have read and understand my rights.

____

Client Signature

____

Date

Appendix 9 - Client Acknowledgements

Below is a sample of a Client Acknowledgement form you might be asked to sign.

Benefits of Neurofeedback

The FDA recognizes that all interventions pose risks and benefits. Typically, the benefits of neurofeedback far outweigh the risks and although on occasion, it can result in non-serious adverse events. As a form of biofeedback, it falls under the category of other low risk activities such as progressive relaxation, hypnosis, breathing exercises, meditation, yoga, and massage. The benefits are usually experienced as improved focus, enhanced concentration, increased energy, higher quality sleep, decreased moodiness, diminished agitation, and reduction in anxiety, as well as reductions in other physical symptoms typically related to stress such as headaches.

Risks of Neurofeedback

Training with neurofeedback can occasionally result in adverse response(s) that temporarily increase symptoms that are typically associated with relaxation and calming of the central nervous system such as fatigue, headaches, lightheadedness, dizziness, irritability, moodiness, weeping, insomnia, agitation, and difficulties with focus and anxiety. These reactions, if they occur, are temporary and typically only last 24–48 hours. Once clients/patients become more relaxed and aware, they tend to integrate past emotional issues and these symptoms subside.

I have participated in a QEEG brain map, have read the notations above, and I would like to pursue neurofeedback training. I understand that:

1. NFB is not a quick fix or cure all, but reduces symptom severity over time through training to improve central nervous system (CNS) regulation.

2. The average number of NFB sessions to achieve enduring change is 40 sessions. This will vary depending on the client/patient's diagnosis, general health, and other factors.

3. On average, most people require 10 - 15 sessions to experience symptom changes. If symptom changes do not occur within 15–20 sessions it is may be due to any one of several factors including but not limited to metabolic conditions, medications, life stress issues, toxins, or a severe medical disorder.

4. Side effects may result from prescribed drugs when dosage is not reduced over sessions which must be guided by the prescribing professional.

5. Some agitation or irritability may occur for a couple of weeks following the 15th session. In some cases, this may not occur while in others onset could occur after only a few sessions. If this occurs, please report this to your neurofeedback practitioner immediately.

6. The chronic use of psychotropic drugs impedes progress.

7. For clients/patients taking psychotropic medications and wanting to reduce or eliminate such; reducing dependence on pharmaceuticals is a key objective of the training program.

8. That client must make efforts to manage diet, exercise, sleep and stressful activities to achieve the best results.

9. Failure to work with practitioners to make lifestyle changes can reduce or mitigate effects of NFB training.

10. Hair analysis or organic acid tests will be required if progress is slow.

11. Clients are expected to complete weekly progress reports the day before their NFB Training sessions. Completion of weekly progress reports helps guide us in providing the best quality of care.

I have read and understand the items outlined above:

________________________________ ______________

Client Signature **Date**

Appendix 10 - Authorization for Release of Information (HIPAA)

Below is a sample of an Authorization for Release of Information form.

Name:________________**Date of Birth**_____ **Client#**___________

(Business Name) is authorized to release protected health information about the above-named individual to the entities named below. The purpose is to inform the professionals or persons listed below in keeping with the patient's instructions.

Entity to Receive Information Check approved to receive information	**Description of information to be released.** Check each that can be given to the person/ entity on the left in the same section.
☐ Voice Mail	☐ Results of QEEG /Assessments ☐ NFB Treatment Sessions ☐ Other
☐ Spouse (provide name & phone number)	☐ Results of QEEG /Assessments ☐ NFB Treatment Sessions ☐ Other
☐ Parent (provide name & phone number)	☐ Results of QEEG /Assessments ☐ NFB Treatment Sessions ☐ Other
☐ Other (provide name & phone number)	☐ Results of QEEG /Assessments ☐ NFB Treatment Sessions ☐ Other
☐ Your E-mail:	☐ Results of QEEG /Assessments ☐ NFB Treatment Sessions ☐ Other
☐ Other E-mail: Name of Person E-mail will go to:	☐ Results of QEEG /Assessments ☐ NFB Treatment Sessions ☐ Other

Personal Information: I understand that I have the right to revoke this authorization at any time and that I have the right to inspect or copy the protected health information to be disclosed as described in this document. I understand that a revocation is not effective in cases where the information has already been disclosed but will be effective going forward.

I understand that information used or disclosed because of this authorization may be subject to redisclosure by the recipient and may no longer be protected by federal or state law.

I understand that I have the right to refuse to sign this authorization and that my treatment will not be conditioned on signing. This authorization shall be in effect until revoked by the individual named above.

____

Signature of Person or Personal Representative

____

Date

Description of Personal Representative's Authority (attach necessary documentation)

Appendix 11 - Financial Policy

Below is a sample of a Financial Policy.

The following information offers some guidelines regarding our financial policy.

We do not take health insurance and are not a Medicaid/Medicare provider.

Please be prepared to pay for services at the time they are rendered.

Please be aware that you are ultimately responsible for the timely payment of your account.

A $35.00 bank fee will be charged for any returned checks.

Past due accounts of 90 days or more may be subject to collections.

Except in cases of emergencies, we require a minimum 24-hour notice if you cannot keep your scheduled appointment. We reserve the right to charge for appointments canceled or broken without a 24-hour notice. Our fee for missed appointments (those without a 24-hour cancellation) is $50.00 per session hour.

For your convenience, we accept cash, personal check, MasterCard, Visa, Discover Card, and American Express.

If you have any questions regarding our policy, please feel free to ask us. We are here to help you!

I have read and agree to the conditions as outlined:

______________________________________ ____________

Client Signature **Date**

Appendix 12 - QEEG Brain Mapping Preparation Checklist

Below is a sample of a QEEG Preparation Checklist you might be given.

The following instructions are for the patient to review and follow before they come in for a QEEG, and will help assure that the best results possible are acquired. **PLEASE PAY ATTENTION to bolded print.**

1. Illness. If you are sick, please call to reschedule even if you only have a cold.

2. Sleep. You should get a good night's sleep before the QEEG. (Let us know if you have any sleep problems or disturbances.)

3. Hair and Scalp. Your hair needs to be clean and dry. Use a pH neutral detergent shampoo such as Neutrogena Anti-Residue or Suave Clarifying shampoo the night before or the on the day of your scheduled appointment. Wash your hair three times. If you have a hair weaves, toupee, or corn-rows, please remove them (if they are removable), before your appointment. No chemical treatments may be administered (coloring, perms, relaxers, etc.) within 48 hours before the QEEG. DO NOT use oils, lotions, mousse, gels, or hairsprays. Hair must be free of beads, weaves, etc. Make sure your hair is completely dry before coming for the QEEG. Please bring a comb or brush.

4. Medications. The QEEG assessment is often cleaner and easier to read if there are no medications in the brain. If the client is taking stimulant medication (i.e., ADHD medication), it is preferable to do the QEEG recording after the patient has stopped taking the medication for up to 48 hours prior.

The client MUST check with his/her prescribing physician or health care provider to determine if it is possible to stop taking the stimulants 48 hours prior to the QEEG. If 48 hours is not advisable, 12–24 is the next preferred length of time. Do not make changes in any other medication(s) unless authorized by your physician. If you are taking medications for anxiety, depression, or sleep, please do NOT stop taking these medications without first consulting with your prescriber.

If you prescriber approves, please bring these medications with you the day of your QEEG and take them after the QEEG assessment has been conducted.

5. Over the Counter Medications and Supplements. Unless prescribed by a physician or licensed health care provider, client should avoid taking any over the counter medication or supplements for 2 or 3 days prior to the QEEG. This includes medications and supplements such as such as: acetaminophen (Tylenol), Advil (Motrin/ibuprofen), aspirin, analgesics, antihistamines/allergy medications (Benadryl, Claritin, Allegra, Zyrtec), cough and cold medicines, herbs, nasal sprays, nutraceuticals (sports drinks, Gatorade, etc.), food supplements (including amino acids), vitamins, or other similar products). If you have any questions about these items, please contact your QEEG practitioner.

6. Caffeinated Beverages. The client should **NOT** drink excessive amounts of coffee, tea, or caffeinated beverages in the morning of the testing (i.e., one cup is fine) and the patient should NOT drink soft drinks with excessive amounts of caffeine in them, i.e., Red Bull, highly caffeinated soft drinks, for at least 15 hours prior to the QEEG.

7. Alcohol and Drugs. Alcohol should be avoided 24 hours prior to your session. Marijuana should be avoided 24–72 hours prior to your session.

8. Contact Lenses. Portions of the QEEG require that your eyes be closed for up to 15 minutes. If you wear contact lenses, please be prepared to remove them if they create discomfort with your eyes closed.

9. Please bring a complete list of medications you take on a daily or regular basis with you when you come for your QEEG.

The day of the QEEG, the client should:

1. Eat a high protein breakfast.
2. Women should not wear any makeup on the forehead or ear lobes.
3. Drink plenty of water the day before the QEEG recording.
4. Use the restroom to prior to the start of the QEEG.
5. No jewelry on neck or ears.
6. Nicotine should be avoided 3 hours prior to your session.
7. Bring any medications or supplements you would like to take after your QEEG is complete.

On the day of your QEEG brain map appointment, plan to spend a minimum of 90 minutes in the office. In addition, you will likely need several minutes to fix your hair following your appointment. Facilities are provided.

PLEASE NOTE: Lack of sleep, medications, low blood sugar, and movement of the eyes, tongue, head or body, may affect the results.

Appendix 13 - Neurofeedback Session Notation Form

Example of neurofeedback session note using SOAP format.

Patient's Name: **ID#:** **Date of service:**

Subjective (client/family report and/or clinical interview data):
Objective: Psychophysiological monitoring using EEG.
Observations:
Impressions/assessment/comments:
Plan:
Protocol name/ID:
Sites A1_ R1 _A1_ G _Cz_ R2 _ A2_ A2_ Threshold
Training Protocol: CH#1 CH#2 Run Length
Seconds # Runs:
Rewards: Multimedia: Station: Vol: Practitioner:
Delta Theta Alpha LoBeta Beta H i B e t a

	Delta	Theta	Aplha	Lo-Beta	Beta	Hi Beta	Hz
Channel 1 Pre							
Channel 1 Post							

Comments:

	Delta	Theta	Aplha	Lo-Beta	Beta	HI Beta	HZ
Channel 2 Pre							
Channel 2 Post							

Comments:
Session # Total Sessions: ____ ____________________
Therapist's Signature

Appendix 14 - Neurofeedback Training Guidelines

Quadrants

Left Front			**Right Front**	
FP1 F3 F7	Delta down Theta down Alpha down Beta up		Fp2 F4 F8	Delta down Theta down Alpha up Beta down
Left Rear			**Right Rear**	
C3 T3 T5 P3 O1	Delta down Theta down Alpha down Beta up		C4 T4 T6 P4 O2	Delta down, Theta down Alpha up Beta down

Midline

Location	Enhance	Inhibit
Fpz		Delta, Theta
Fz	SMR, Beta	Delta, Theta
Cz	SMR	Delta, Theta
Pz	Theta, Alpha	Delta

Appendix 15 - Drug Effects on EEG

Family	Drugs	Purpose	EEG Impact
Neuroleptics	Haldol, Prolixin, Thorazine, Mellaril	sedative	increase delta, theta and beta above 20 Hz and decrease alpha and beta below 20 Hz.
Neuroleptics	Seroquel, Risperdal, Geodone	non-sedative &antipsychotic medications	decrease alpha and increase beta in general.
Anxiolytics	Valium, Halcion, Librium, Dalmane	anxiety relief	decrease alpha and increase beta, especially 13-20 Hz beta
Benzodiazepines	Valium, Xanax, and Ativan	anxiety, panic relief	decrease alpha and increase 20-30 Hz beta
SSRIs	Prozac, Paxil, and Zoloft	a class of antidepressants used in the treatment of depression, anxiety disorders, and some personality disorders.	decrease in frontal alpha and a mild increase in 18-25 Hz beta.
MAO Inhibitors	Marplan, Parnate, Eldepryl	antidepressant	tendency to increase 20-30 Hz beta while decreasing all other frequencies

Tricyclic antidepressants	Imipramine and Amitriptyline	useful in depressed patients with insomnia, restlessness, and nervousness	increase delta and theta while decreasing alpha; increase beta 25 Hz and up band
Antipsychotics	Lithium	used for the treatment of manic/depressive (bipolar) and depressive disorders	increases theta, mildly decreases alpha and increases beta
Amphetamines	Adderall, Vyvanse, and Dexedrine.	a group of drugs that act by increasing levels of norepinephrine, serotonin, and dopamine in the brain	decrease slow-wave activity and increase beta in the 12-26 Hz range
Marijuana		recreational	increases frontal low frequency alpha; affects EEG for three days
Opiates	opium, hydromorphone, oxymorphone, heroin, morphine, oxycodone, Talwin, codeine, methadone, meperdine	pain relief	pain relief generate high amplitude slow alpha in the 8 Hz range
Barbiturates	Brevital, thiamylal (Surital), thiopental (Pentothal), amobarbital, Amytal, pentobarbital,	produce a wide spectrum of central nervous system depression, from mild sedation to coma, and have been used as sedatives, hypnotics, anesthetics, and anticonvulsants	increase beta at 25-35 Hz amplitude

Appendix 16 – Sample Mentoring Documentation Form

Name:
Technician:
Office Phone:
Session:

Date:
Equipment:
Cell Phone:
Consult Type:
Consult Fee:

Concepts/Applications Reviewed

- ☐ qEEG Interpretation
- ☐ Power/Magnitude
- ☐ Phase
- ☐ Coherence
- ☐ Dominant Frequency
- ☐ Asymmetry
- ☐ Discriminants
- ☐ Remapping
- ☐ Identifying Artifacts
- ☐ Editing qEEG Record
- ☐ Montages
- ☐ Managing EMG

- ☐ Interpreting Trend Screens
- ☐ Setting Thresholds & Auto-thresholding
- ☐ Interpreting Z scores

- ☐ Training File Management
- ☐ Using Psychometrics
- ☐ Tracking Symptoms

- ☐ Session Profile & Management
- ☐ Paste & Connections

- ☐ Protocol Determination
- ☐ Protocol Evaluation
- ☐ Changing Protocols
- ☐ Training Landmarks
- ☐ Remapping Criteria
- ☐ Progress Review
- ☐ Managing Client Expectations
- ☐ Explain NFB To Clients
- ☐ Client Coaching

Case 1

Client Initials:	Age:
Gender:	Follow Up:
Dx:	
Map Type:	Pwr:
Dom Freq:	Coher:
Asym Alpha:	Asym Beta:
Protocol 1#	Protocol 2#:
Session #:	Session #:
Location	Location

Change Re Norm
New Protocol #: Location

Comments:

Case 2

Client Initials:	Age:
Gender:	Follow Up:
Dx:	
Map Type:	Pwr:
Dom Freq:	Coher:
Asym Alpha:	Asym Beta:
Protocol 1#	Protocol 2#:
Session #:	Session #:
Location	Location

Change Re Norm
New Protocol #: Location

Comments:

www.ingramcontent.com/pod-product-compliance
Lightning Source LLC
Chambersburg PA
CBHW071138280326
41935CB00010B/1273

* 9 7 8 0 9 9 7 8 1 9 4 5 8 *